$\mathcal{P}$REGNANCY MYTHS

$\mathcal{A}$n OBSTETRICIAN
DEMYSTIFIES PREGNANCY
from CONCEPTION TO BIRTH

Combines two volumes:
Pregnancy Myths
and
Birth Day!
The Last 24 Hours of Pregnancy

MICHAEL D. BENSON, M.D.

MARLOWE & COMPANY
NEW YORK

Published by
Marlowe & Company
841 Broadway, Fourth Floor
New York, NY 10003

Pregnancy Myths: An Obstetrician Demystifies Pregnancy from Conception to Birth combines two previously published volumes:

Pregnancy Myths
Copyright © 1995 by Michael D. Benson

Birth Day! The Last 24 Hours of Pregnancy
Copyright © 1993 by Michael D. Benson

Library of Congress Cataloging-in-Publication Data

Benson, Michael D.
    Pregnancy myths : an obstretrician demystifies
pregnancy from conception to birth / Michael D. Benson.
      p.   cm.
    Includes index.
    ISBN 1-56924-695-5
    Pregnancy—Miscellanea. 2. Childbirth—Miscellanea. 3.
Labor (Obstetrics)—Popular works. 4. Childbirth—
Popular works.
    I. Title.
    RG525.B464   1998
    618.2'4—dc 21   98-28523
                                       CIP

Manufactured in the United States of America

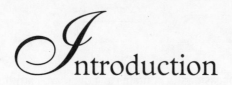

Introduction

Trends and Issues in Childbirth Education

Several trends over the past 20 years have changed the way doctors and medical staff relate to pregnant women—both in terms of education and medical care. Perhaps the most important trend has been patients' greater awareness of consumer advocacy issues. Women now ask for more explanation and information about their illnesses and possible treatments. The old standby among doctors, "Because I said so," simply won't work. While this response had been more or less accepted in the first half of this century, no patient today would find it acceptable.

Medicine itself has also changed with increasing emphasis on science and technology. While this has permitted physicians to treat more illnesses successfully, it has also served to make treatment less personal and more difficult to understand. Other changes in medicine include an expanded list of ethical issues that must be dealt with and a need for improved doctor-patient communications.

As an obstetrician in private practice, I regularly encourage my patients to read more about childbirth and attend education classes. However, in written material as well as in classes, the information conveyed is sometimes either simply not true or is presented with a lack of perspective that serves to mislead. In fact, the material presented occasionally contains an adversarial attitude toward doctors, nurses, and hospital personnel. In an effort to give women more and better information, I have written two books, *Pregnancy Myths* and *Birth Day! The Last 24 Hours of Pregnancy*, which have been combined here into one volume.

This text has a more ambitious purpose than merely to educate. It is intended to broaden the reader's perspective and provide a foundation for better communication with health care personnel. To this end, the five major issues noted below have an important impact on the patient-physician relationship.

Patients' independence in decision making is a concept that is receiving increasing emphasis in medical school curricula. In medical parlance it is also known as patient autonomy. It refers to the idea that patients as much as possible should be free to make their own decisions about treatment—even if they may be "bad" choices. In theory, a patient who is writhing in pain and quite sick from a ruptured appendix should be free to decline surgery even though this decision results in a very poor outcome. Of course, the concept of autonomy can lead to some very real practical problems. Is such a patient truly in his or her right mind (i.e. legally competent to choose)? Will the estate of the deceased patient hold the physician responsible for failing to intervene? Though this example of the problems raised by patient autonomy may seem far removed from daily concerns, in fact, the physician and patient's autonomy have very real implications for both the way the parties communicate and their expectations.

I can recall having a conversation with one patient who was being scheduled for a minor surgical procedure. She had expressed fear about going to sleep. When I offered her the choice of staying awake with a spinal anesthetic or going to sleep with a general anesthetic, she became quite upset and stormed out of the office. She thought "How can I go to a doctor who does not know what type of anesthesia I should have?" While this is an extreme example, many patients actually feel most comfortable when the doctor picks their option for them and makes all the treatment decisions.

Often there is no right or wrong position to take. It is helpful for patients to know which style of care they prefer and whom they prefer to make treatment decisions—the doctor or themselves. It is worth remembering, however, that the physician may not be equally comfortable in either mode. Some prefer to make the decisions themselves while other doctors feel that patient autonomy is an overriding objective and that patients should choose.

Although I feel comfortable in either mode, I believe that an important challenge of medical practice is to figure out what style the patient prefers. It is not always easy, particularly when patients are not aware of their own preferences. I always like to give treatment options although I am usually careful to rank them in order of desirability. Nonetheless, patients will occasionally be confused and uncertain even when I explain why option A is better than options B, C, or D. In these cases, I sometimes suggest "If you are in doubt or confused, my advice is to follow my advice."

Informed consent is another concept that has assumed increasing importance in the past several decades. Related to the idea of patient autonomy, it requires that patients are fully informed of the risks, benefits, limitations, and alternatives to a given treatment before agreeing to the treatment. Unfortunately, in practice the idea has definite limits. What laboring mother can truly give "informed consent" when the doctor (correctly or incorrectly) advises an emergency Cesarean section because the fetus is in immediate jeopardy? Everyone feels that they made a good decision when the medical treatment works well and has no ill effect; yet no one feels that they made a good decision when they are one of the unlucky ones to sustain a complication.

It would be remiss of me not to mention the oppressive **threat of lawsuits** in connection with patient and physician communication. This is perhaps one reason why many obstetricians simply provide a blanket statement that no medication or prescription is completely safe to take during pregnancy. This is neither scientifically accurate nor good advice, but many obstetricians feel that they can be sued if a patient takes a medication and coincidentally delivers a child with a birth defect. In our practice, we attempt to ignore the threat of litigation and simply provide the best treatment we can. Nonetheless, the fear that a physician's own words can be used against him or her in an adversarial environment can hinder open communication with patients.

A fourth issue that comes up in patient education programs or doctor-patient communications is the **lack of patients' technical information**. This can make explaining certain illnesses, treatments, or lab tests very difficult when the ideas involved are abstract and outside of daily experience. For instance, a blood test for birth defects such as Down's Syndrome is calculated and reported in a way very unfamiliar to most patients. Typically the test will report a risk of having an afflicted child such as 1 in 79. Of course, patients want to know what "normal" is. The only reasonable answer is that normal is the less than 1 in 200. This level comes from the risk of causing a miscarriage with amniocentesis—the procedure required to establish whether or not the fetus really has Down's syndrome. Yet to most patients, this explanation makes no sense since the test report is unlike anything they have encountered before.

Finally, patient education and communication can be limited simply because science does not have all the answers. Imagine an eighteenth-century physician trying to explain pneumonia or syphilis before bacteria were discovered. Many symptoms and aspects of pregnancy simply are not understood. For instance, we have no idea of what causes morning sickness or why labor starts when it does. What's worse, some of the things that we thought we knew turned out to be wrong. For instance, mental retardation and cerebral palsy were formerly believed to be due to lack of oxygen during labor. We know now that this is the exception rather than the rule.

With these ideas in mind, I have undertaken to write about two aspects of pregnancy: widely-held myths, and the last day of pregnancy which is filled with labor and is probably the single most anxiety-provoking day of the entire nine months. This book is intended to do more than merely entertain or inform. My hope is that it will give perspective to pregnant women to allow them to discern for themselves the boundaries between myth, fact, and opinion.

All five of the issues mentioned above are addressed in some manner in the two books.

1. Independence in decision making. The material provided here seeks to give the reader a broad foundation on which she can base decisions. Though not every situation can be anticipated, the ideas of scientific testing, relative risk, and the boundaries between the known and unknown can help patients choose rationally when choices in treatment exist.

2. Informed consent. By addressing the common issues that arise in labor well in advance, the reader will be in a better position to judge the risks and benefits of a specific treatment even in circumstances of pain and/or anxiety.

3. Practicing defensive medicine due to the pervasive fear of malpractice. One manifestation of defensive medicine, "do not take any medicine at all during pregnancy," is specifically debunked in *Pregnancy Myths*. Other bits of defensive advice are also examined.

4. Lack of technical background of most patients. While these books provide some medical/technical background, they obviously cannot provide all the technical information a woman undergoing treatment might need in order to judge the course of action being recommended. But I believe they go a long way toward providing enough technical knowledge so that the patient will be able to view the medical decisions being made in better perspective.

5. The limits of scientific knowledge. Perhaps most important of all, readers will develop a sensitivity to distinguishing established fact from care-giver opinion. While I try to distinguish between what I believe may be true and what is scientifically established as true, not all health-care providers feel equally comfortable in making such issues clear. Sometimes the difference can be crucial. With the approach taken here, it is hoped that readers will acquire an improved sense that will allow them to discern the different degrees of scientific certainty.

The first portion of this book, *Pregnancy Myths*, is dedicated to the belief that knowledge empowers. The anxiety caused by myths and incorrect facts can be addressed by critical examination. With a skeptical view of 100 or so widely believed but untrue ideas, *Pregnancy Myths* seeks both to entertain and to restore common sense to the dos and don'ts of pregnancy.

The second part, *Birth Day*, addresses the anxiety of every pregnant woman: **What will my labor be like?** Topics such as LaMaze breathing, pain medication, episiotomy, and Cesarean section are examined in detail. The time course of labor and hospital routine are also explained so that every woman facing labor should have some idea of what to expect. Such knowledge can help pregnant women to better understand and choose among the options they face during labor.

Finally, although these books describe what is commonly done or experienced, they are no substitute for the advice and insights of your health-care giver. As the obstetrician who wrote these books, I do not handle a given clinical situation the same way every time. The practice of medicine truly remains an art as well as a science. With this in mind, these books are intended to serve as guide to what can be or may be done and experienced during pregnancy and childbirth. It can hardly be considered a standard of care, as I prefer to individualize care for a specific patient rather than simply follow the rules of a medical text "cookbook" that will not necessarily be appropriate for all patients. Certainly, other obstetricians have their own ways of doing things.

A word of practical advice: Whenever your anxiety keeps you awake at night, call your doctor. If you are in doubt about whether you should call, call. One of the biggest services that we as obstetricians can provide is emotional support.

Michael D. Benson, MD, FACOG
February, 1998
Deerfield, Illinois

$\mathscr{C}$ontents of Pregnancy Myths

Preparing for and Predicting Labor

MYTHS:

CHAPTER FOUR: *Childbirth*

The Amniotic Membranes

MYTHS:

Cesarean Delivery

MYTHS:

CHAPTER FIVE: *The Baby Before, During, and After Birth*

Gender Prediction

MYTHS:

Fetal Health

MYTHS:

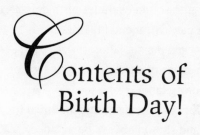

Contents of Birth Day!

PREGNANCY
MYTHS

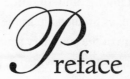

Preface

My patients have been the inspiration for this book, for none of the myths that are included here are of academic straw men. These have been actual concerns or beliefs of the many women who come to me for medical advice or treatment. I am happy to report that in talking to them I have been successful in debunking most, but not all, of the myths contained in this book. Sometimes people cling to mistaken ideas with great fervor.

In the crowded literature of pregnancy and childbirth, it is no mean trick to come up with a topic that has not been previously covered. Yet, with all the fallacies, mistaken notions, and simple falsehoods—both in the spoken and printed word—it is remarkable that a book cataloging these "myths" has not already been published.

This book is intended to serve two purposes. First, it is meant to counter dozens of mistaken notions concerning pregnancy. Second, it is hoped that these examples will help the general population become more skeptical and analytical when it comes to all medically related information. The subject of "health" is widely targeted by writers with varying qualifications, and all too often, with the primary objective of scaring their audience.

There are hundreds of professional or scientific publications relating to Obstetrics and Gynecology. As new studies are published, the understanding and practice of clinical medicine changes. This change, as predictable as the seasons, is an inherent and permanent feature of the summary sources cited above. While most of facts and perspectives provided in this book are not likely to change, some of them may as new information becomes available.

I have made every effort to adhere to a high standard of accuracy. Yet try as I may, I cannot guarantee that all statements in this book are absolutely true and represent the last word on the subjects in question. Statements presented as fact are what the author understands to be the consensus medical view at the time of publication. As such, these statements do not represent a unanimous view, and even the consensus medical view can change over time. It is ultimately up to the reader to decide their soundness and currency. Yet where this book takes on specific myths that have been studied by medical researchers in some depth, the weight of the medical evidence leaves little room for doubt.

Michael D. Benson, M.D., F.A.C.O.G.

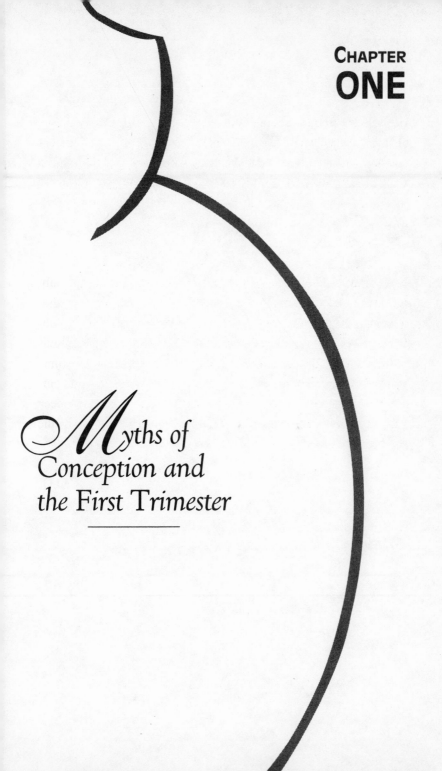

Myths of
Conception and
the First Trimester

High Risk

MYTH #1:

A pregnant woman age 35 or over is at "high risk."

This misleading idea weaves together a number of thin strands of truth. It is true that the incidence of illness increases with age and that the percentage of birth defects increases with a mother's age. However, the conclusion that becoming pregnant at 35 or over is dangerous and likely to produce a sick or abnormal child is simply wrong. To understand why, it is necessary to look at the concept of "risk," the relationship between maternal age and health, and the link between maternal age and fetal well-being in closer detail.

The concept of "high risk" pregnancy was developed in the 1960s as researchers began to examine large data bases on pregnant women in an effort to predict in advance which individual pregnancies were at risk for bad outcomes. It was hoped that mothers identified as being at "high risk"—either for injury to themselves or for giving birth to sick infants—could be helped through modifications in their prenatal care. Unfortunately, this so-called global risk scoring for bad outcomes has not proven too useful because it identifies a large minority of women as "high risk," while relatively few of these patients have bad outcomes. Also, simply identifying a patient as being at higher-than-average risk for any type of bad result is less useful than specifying the particular danger so that preventive measures can be individualized. In current practice, obstetricians tend to focus more on specific dangers for a given patient rather than simply making a general assessment of risk. For instance, increased risk of having a birth defect includes diabetes and maternal age, while risk factors for preterm birth include multiple gestations, maternal smoking, or a prior history of preterm birth. In view of the limited utility of global risk scoring, the term "high risk" is too vague to have much meaning.

It is true that the risk of maternal illness and death increases with advancing age. However, death remains so uncommon even in older age groups that it is misleading to cite this fact to prospective parents. For instance, the death rate per 100,000 women has been estimated at approximately 15 for women between the age of 20–24 and rises to 58 in those aged 35–39. While this four-fold increase may seem impressive, out of every 10,000 older women, 9,995 will survive the pregnancy. For perspective, one to two of these 10,000 women will die in the year of their pregnancy from auto accidents (yet all of us still drive). It is also important to recognize that, in the real world, reaching the age of 35 does not signal a sudden increase in risk. The maternal mortality rate rises steadily, and these specific ages do not represent some sudden form of biological deterioration.

Some authors also make much of the fact that maternal illnesses, such as diabetes and hypertension are more common in older pregnant women. While this is true, these patients would have these maladies whether they became pregnant or not. In general, with proper medical care, these conditions can be quite readily treated, resulting in a happy outcome for mother and baby.

What about fetal well-being in pregnancies of older women? The stillbirth rate and poor neonatal outcome among older pregnant patients has been shown in several studies to be no different than in younger women. As a group, older women are more likely to be married, college-educated, and financially secure—factors thought to play a major role in good pregnancy outcomes.

One oft-cited concern for older women is that of birth defects. Approximately 3 percent of newborns have any sort of birth defect. About 20 percent of these problems belong to a specific group of disorders known as chromosome abnormalities. All of us have 46 chromosomes (individual collections of thousands of genes). Those who have extra or missing chromosome material commonly have major problems such as mental retardation and anatomical abnormalities. Most pregnancies with chromosome abnormalities end in miscarriage or fetal demise. Among those babies with chromosome abnormalities that are live-born, Down's syndrome (an extra number 21 chromosome) is the most common. Chromosome abnormalities are the only group of birth defects known to increase with maternal age. These birth defects can be detected by amniocentesis in which a needle is placed through the abdominal wall and fluid containing fetal cells is withdrawn from around the fetus.

What does this mean for older women? At age 20, the risk for having a live-born infant with a chromosome error is approximately one in 526. At age 30 it is one in 384. By age 34 it rises to one in 243, and at age 35, it is one in 178. For a mother who is 40 at the time of delivery, the risk goes up to one in 63. Even for this older woman, the chance that she will NOT have a baby with a chromosome error is 62 out of 63, or 98.4 percent.

The risk of causing a miscarriage from the amniocentesis is thought to be on the order of one in 200. Recalling the risks cited above, it can be seen that delivery at the maternal age of 35 is the first age at which the chance of finding a problem through amniocentesis exceeds the risk of causing a problem by doing the test. With this reasoning, it has been common practice the world over to recommend amniocentesis to women who will be age 35 and over on their due date. It is worth pointing out that of 178 women who are 35 at the time of birth, only one will have a child with a chromosome error.

In summary, the term "high risk" is so vague that it no longer has much meaning. While it is true that the maternal death rate rises with age, this event remains so uncommon among older women that it should not be a major concern. Babies born to older women appear to be just as healthy as those born to younger mothers. The one thing that is done differently for pregnant women age 35 and over is that they are routinely offered amniocentesis due to the slightly increased risk of chromosome abnormalities (like Down's syndrome). However, as can be seen, this type of birth defect remains unlikely even in the babies of older women. Women do not suddenly deteriorate at age 35. With the exception of amniocentesis, older women are not treated any differently during their prenatal care.

The Due Date

MYTH #2:
The due date is determined from the time of conception.

The due date is initially assigned at 40 weeks past the first day of the last menstrual period. This assignment is based on the assumption that conception occurred on cycle day 14, which it does typically in women with 28-day cycles. Many of my patients will perceptively point out, "But I'm not even pregnant during the first two weeks of your pregnancy calculations!" This is, of course, quite true. For perspective, it is worth remembering that estimating the time of the baby's arrival on the basis of the last menstrual period has been practiced for thousands of years. The concept of ovulation, by comparison, is relatively new—only a century or so old. Right or wrong, when the medical literature (or patient charting for that matter) refers to gestational age, it invariably refers to a time scale that begins with the first day of the last period. This terminology for describing gestational age is even used when there is no meaningful last period such as when a woman becomes pregnant while nursing.

By definition, the due date is the midpoint of when the baby is expected. Ninety percent of pregnancies will end with labor within two weeks either way from this date. Roughly 5 percent of pregnancies will deliver more than two weeks in advance and are thus premature, while 5 percent will deliver more than 14 days after the due date and are thereby postmature. Health problems for the fetus can arise from either of these extremes.

MYTH #3:
The due date established by ultrasound is more accurate than the due date established by the last menstrual period.

Ultrasounds can assign due dates during the first 24 weeks of pregnancy because fetuses do not show much genetic variation in size. As a result, by measuring fetal structures to the nearest millimeter, doctors can arrive at fairly good estimates of gestational age. These measurements are not so precise, nor are babies so uniform, that size assessment in the first two trimesters of pregnancies is perfect in assigning a due date. As a general rule, if the ultrasound-assigned due date agrees to within seven days of the menstrual-period due date, the original due date is not changed. However, because ultrasound is a relatively costly procedure and also produces a picture, many patients assume that the due date is more reliable than a guesstimate that took five seconds for the doctor to produce. Not so. Also, ultrasounds done in the last 12 weeks of pregnancy are not useful in predicting the baby's arrival. Genetic variation begins to cause babies of the same age to vary in size by this time. The rule, which works earlier in the pregnancy when size is closely related to age, no longer applies.

MYTH #4:
Women who have had in-vitro fertilization know exactly when labor will occur.

This idea never occurred to me until one of our patients who had in-vitro fertilization expressed puzzlement as to why she had not delivered on her due date. Her confusion was logical enough since she actually knew the hour in which conception occurred. Nonetheless, it is not known in humans whether the labor cascade is started by maternal or fetal events. (In sheep, it is the fetus.) As a result, while in-vitro fertilization patients know their due date with a very high degree of precision, the actual start of labor remains speculative. As with women with less high-tech conceptions, almost half the babies will deliver before the due date and about half will deliver after.

Miscarriage

MYTH #5:

Cramping in early pregnancy is a warning signal for miscarriage.

Many patients have heard or read that "cramping is a warning signal for miscarriage." In addition, a great number of pregnant women in my practice complain of menstrual-type cramping or even achiness on one side or the other in the lower abdomen. Despite its apparent frequency in the first trimester, such cramping and lower abdominal pain without vaginal bleeding is rarely if ever mentioned in the medical literature.

In my view, based on personal observation, this mild discomfort should be considered normal and not predictive of illness. However, a critical distinction must be made between those who have "cramping" without bleeding and those who have "cramping" with bleeding. Those women who have bleeding, whether or not they have any pelvic discomfort, may subsequently miscarry. In the absence of bleeding, mild cramping or achiness is simply not worrisome. As always is the case, severe pain (whether crampy or not) should be brought to a physician's attention.

MYTH #6:

**Cramping in early pregnancy is an indication that
an ectopic pregnancy has occurred.**

An ectopic pregnancy is a pregnancy in which the fertilized egg implants and grows outside the appropriate portion of the uterus or womb. Among the inappropriate locations to grow, the embryo most frequently implants within the Fallopian tube, thus the synonymous name, tubal pregnancy. Unfortunately, the tubal structure and blood supply are not sufficient to sustain a pregnancy so that these embryos are invariably doomed to miscarry. They also pose a special threat to the pregnant woman because they can cause substantial internal bleeding as they are expelled from the tube back into the abdominal cavity. On occasion, the pregnancy can momentarily thrive and actually burst the tube, causing significant pain and life-threatening internal bleeding.

Some of my patients have told me that they have read that cramping can be a symptom of a tubal pregnancy. Certainly such a belief would disturb any pregnant woman who happened to have such cramps. The fact is that tubal pregnancies are uncommon, occurring in perhaps one out of every 100 pregnancies. While it is correct that the vast majority of patients who have an ectopic pregnancy have abdominal pain as one of their symptoms, the reverse is not true. Most pregnant women who have pain in the first trimester do not have anything wrong with their pregnancy. This is particularly true for those with mild cramping reminiscent of menstrual cramps and mild degrees of dull achiness. On the other hand, pain with bleeding, increasing pain, or pain that interferes with normal activities warrants discussion with a physician.

Myth #7:
Vigorous exercise increases the risk of miscarriage.

Exercise is not thought to be a cause of miscarriage. While the cause of many miscarriages is not known, the leading reason that we know of is a genetic abnormality of the embryo. It is worth pointing out that a pregnant woman cannot "shake the baby loose" any more than she can shake her kidney or intestines loose. Exercise simply does not generate the force necessary cause the embryo to separate from the uterus. Even the rise in body temperature generated in vigorous exercise is not thought to result in any embryonic harm.

Myth #8:
Falling can cause miscarriages.

In a memorable scene from *Gone With the Wind,* Scarlet O'Hara and Rhett Butler are arguing at the top of their grand staircase when he nudges her and she accidentally falls down the entire flight of stairs. It does not help their marriage when she promptly miscarries as a result. Yet, in truth, a maternal fall will not result in miscarriage unless it is so violent that she needs immediate hospitalization and surgery for rupture of internal organs.

In normal pregnancies, the embryo is firmly attached to the wall of the uterus and considerable force directed at the uterus itself is required to cause a separation of the developing pregnancy from the maternal tissues. These forces would be generally sufficient to cause other pelvic organs to separate from their attachments, necessitating emergency surgery even for nonpregnant women. Maternal trauma is not even discussed in the medical literature as a cause of miscarriage except to dismiss it.

Myth #9:
A woman who miscarries always (or never) needs a D and C.

Perhaps a word on terminology is in order here. The medical profession, by tradition, refers to any pregnancy cessation in the first half of pregnancy as an "abortion." Of course, this term is very distressing to those women who lose desired pregnancies. In this context, acts of nature will be designated as "miscarriages" in keeping with the lay person's terminology. Also, the term D and C, a reference to dilation and curettage, is not precisely correct here. When performed in a pregnant patient, the procedure is known as a D and E for dilation and evacuation, or a suction curettage. The unique feature of this procedure done in pregnancy is the use of the suction curette, a hollow plastic tube through which a vacuum is created, facilitating removal of the pregnancy tissue.

A "threatened" miscarriage is a reference to vaginal bleeding in the first trimester in the absence of cervical dilation or the passage of tissue. An "inevitable" miscarriage is defined as vaginal bleeding in the presence of cervical dilation. In practice, this can only be diagnosed by physical examination of the cervix. This condition typically lasts for only a few hours at the most and is usually accompanied by heavy bleeding and cramping. A "missed" miscarriage is a pregnancy in which the embryo is known to be nonviable, but has not yet been expelled from the body. The nonviability of the pregnancy can be established through ultrasound or dropping serial quantitative HCG's. (This is the pregnancy hormone, human chorionic gonadotropin, which is measured in pregnancy tests. Falling levels in early pregnancy suggest embryonic demise.) An "incomplete" miscarriage occurs when part of the pregnancy tissue has been expelled and some remains within the uterus.

A suction curettage generally is appropriate in three situations. For those women who have bleeding and cramping and also have a dilated cervix (i.e., an inevitable miscarriage), a D and E can save them several hours of bleeding and pain. This is also true for those who have had an incomplete miscarriage. When it has been determined that the embryo is dead, but it and the products of conception have not yet been expelled, a suction curettage can bring closure to the process as well as prevent hours of bleeding and cramping later on.

Suction curettages for miscarriages are rarely medical "necessities." They should be viewed as largely elective procedures to alleviate the pain and bleeding of the actual miscarriage process. For women determined to do so, a suction curettage can be avoided by simply putting up with the discomfort of expelling the pregnancy. Of course, the duration, amount of pain, and volume of bleeding vary from woman to woman. Also, the longer the pregnancy has progressed until embryonic demise, the more uncomfortable the process.

There are two uncommon circumstances in which the suction curettage is necessary to prevent a significant threat to health. In rare cases, the miscarriage process can result in life-threatening bleeding. Also, when weeks have passed since embryonic demise, the pregnancy tissue can become infected within the uterus. It is worth emphasizing that these are very unusual events, and in most cases, the suction curettage is recommended to alleviate suffering in contrast to preventing a life-threatening condition.

MYTH #10:
Hormone imbalances are a common cause of miscarriages.

Virtually everyone who miscarries wants to know why. Unfortunately, doctors often have little explanation to offer other than "the sperm and the egg did not unite properly." From this void has emerged the idea that a progesterone deficiency is a common reason for pregnancy failure. After ovulation, the ovary produces progesterone, which is thought to sustain the pregnancy until about eight weeks' gestation, at which time the placenta itself takes over progesterone production. It is well established that removing the ovary from which ovulation took place early in a pregnancy will result in a miscarriage. It also seems likely that a very few women have an inherent biological abnormality in which an ovary does not produce satisfactory amounts of progesterone, resulting in infertility or repetitive early miscarriage.

With patients exerting pressure to find (and fix) the cause of miscarriage, many doctors have resorted to prescribing progesterone suppositories in early pregnancy. Unfortunately, there seems to be no scientific basis for doing this since progesterone deficiencies are thought to be rare. To make the issue more confusing, a low progesterone level is actually a sign that the pregnancy itself is not normal—not that the ovary is inherently defective and unable to produce enough progesterone to sustain a pregnancy. In other words, measuring progesterone levels in early pregnancy cannot diagnose progesterone deficiencies. To the extent it can be diagnosed, it is done by doing testing in a nonpregnant menstrual cycle. Although progesterone suppositories are actually made of the same progesterone molecule already produced by the body, the safety of this intervention is not absolutely known. It is widely believed to be at least harmless (if not helpful).

MYTH #11:

A woman who miscarries is actually fortunate because the baby would have been abnormal.

While it is true that a common cause of miscarriage is some profound genetic defect of the embryo (i.e., a chromosome error such as Down's syndrome), few women who miscarry feel "lucky." They are not thankful that they did not carry a baby with a birth defect; rather they wonder why they did not have a healthy baby as their friend, relative, or neighbor did. In trying to console someone who has had an early pregnancy loss, it would be best to avoid saying, "It was meant to be," or "You're really lucky because the baby would have been abnormal." A more appropriate condolence would be "I'm sorry for your loss," or "I know this is a sad time for you."

Early Symptoms

MYTH #12:
Wrist bands alleviate morning sickness.

There are commercially available wrist bands that are promoted to control motion sickness through "acupressure." Occasionally pregnant women will try these devices to control pregnancy-associated nausea as well. I could find no reference in the medical literature to this practice; apparently it has not been studied. The manufacturer of one such device that I checked on made no claims as to its efficacy based on medical studies. The fairest statement that can be made is that wrist pressure, used to reduce the nausea during pregnancy, is not known *or* suspected to be effective.

MYTH #13:
Women with severe morning sickness are trying to "vomit out the pregnancy."

Ironically, the first time I ever heard this myth was from an obstetrician, although I have no doubt many lay people believe it as well. Of interest is the fact that medical texts do cite studies in which stress was believed to play a significant role in the occurrence of morning sickness. On the other hand, some studies seem to show a relationship between either the absolute amount of pregnancy hormone in the maternal bloodstream or its rate of rise. In general, this phenomenon is poorly understood, and there does not seem to be a consensus in the medical literature on why it occurs in some pregnancies and not in others.

Based on my personal observations of pregnant women with and without nausea, it is my belief that this symptom is a result of biochemistry that is not yet understood. For example, perhaps some pregnancies produce a nausea-causing protein while others do not. While this is entirely speculative, it seems fair to say that the cause of nausea in pregnancy is not well understood. Nausea is commonly experienced to a mild degree by most pregnant women, but we do not know why some women have absolutely no symptoms and others are afflicted so severely that they lose weight. Suggesting that a pregnant woman's severe nausea is due to the fact that she does not want the pregnancy sounds to me like blaming the victim.

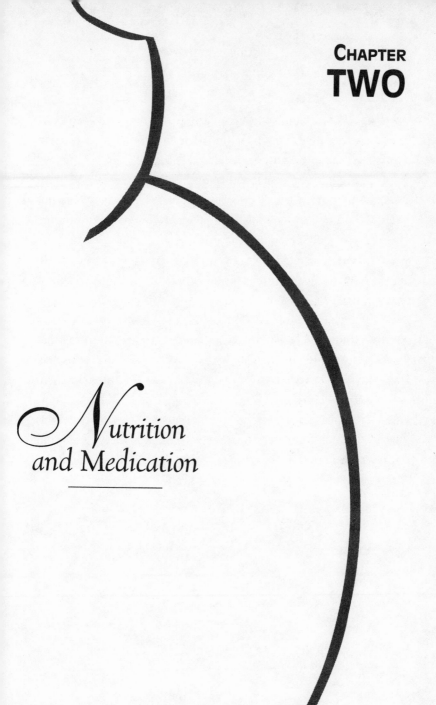

Nutrition
and Medication

Diet

MYTH #14:

Fruit juice is the drink of choice for a pregnant woman.

A s I tell many patients, "If Einstein were alive today and starting a new career, he might well be tempted to take up marketing." After all, many of our creative geniuses seem to be working in this field. The mistaken notion that one should drink a lot of fruit juice during pregnancy is surely responsible for many tons of excess weight gain in pregnant women across the country every year.

When I checked the nutrition labeling on the carton of orange juice in my refrigerator, several facts become clear. It has 110 calories in eight ounces and no fat or protein. Coca-Cola Classic in comparison has only 96 calories in eight ounces. A single orange has only about 65 calories, or roughly half the calories of a glass of juice. The only nutrient that the juice has in substantial amounts is vitamin C. As will be seen later in the myth concerning vitamins, pregnant women (and nonpregnant people) should be getting enough vitamin C in their diet already as long as they are eating three meals a day.

It has been estimated that 3,500 calories are required to produce a pound of fat in the body. With this in mind, what are the consequences of a pregnant woman deciding to drink two glasses of juice a day instead of the two glasses of water? She would be adding 220 calories per day to her diet. Assuming a pregnancy of 280 days, this would amount to 61,600 calories over the course of the entire pregnancy or an estimated 17.6 pounds. This is a lot of weight from juice alone. Any pregnant woman concerned about excess weight gain should eliminate fruit juice entirely from her diet. It is not a good substitute for fruit. While this example may oversimplify the relationship of calorie intake to weight gain, it is worth remembering that even a moderate daily increase in calorie consumption can add 10 to 20 unwanted pounds over the course of a pregnancy.

MYTH #15:
Nutrasweet is not safe for pregnant women.

This is not just a myth in our overweight society, but a dangerous fallacy. Nutrasweet is not only safe for pregnant women, it is much safer than sugar, a so-called natural component of our diet! Since this statement is not intuitive and a direct challenge to the New Age "everything should be natural" thinking, it is well worth explaining.

Nutrasweet is the brand name of aspartame, a modified combination of two naturally occurring amino acids: phenylalanine and aspartic acid. Amino acids are the building blocks of proteins much like letters are used to form words. Just as there are 26 letters in the English language, there are 20 amino acids from which human proteins are made. Aspartame is 200 times sweeter than sucrose, a naturally occurring sugar. Its property of sweetness was discovered accidentally in 1965 by a chemist working for the pharmaceutical company Searle.

Aspartame is processed by the body much as any protein would be. Its digestion results in three breakdown products: aspartic acid, phenylalanine, and methanol. It has been estimated that the average aspartic acid intake in young adults is roughly 170 milligrams per kilogram of body weight. If an individual entirely replaced sugar intake with an equivalent sweetness dose of aspartame, aspartic acid intake would increase by approximately 5 milligrams per kilogram of body weight. This represents roughly a 2 percent increase in the consumption of a naturally occurring substance already in our diet. It is hard to imagine how this could pose any sort of health threat to anyone, pregnant or not.

Aspartic acid levels can be directly measured in the bloodstream. In studies of human metabolism of aspartame, doses that yield 13 mg/kg of aspartic acid were found to cause no significant change in blood levels of this amino acid for 24 hours after ingestion. Even at exceedingly high levels of intake (200 mg/kg), aspartic acid levels were found to be less elevated than after a normal adult meal.

Phenylalanine is a second breakdown product of aspartame. This, too, is an amino acid that is a vital and naturally occurring component of our diet. The same types of data acquired for aspartic acid also proved to apply to phenylalanine—normal adults simply did not experience a significant rise in their blood levels with any conceivably possible dose of aspartame. However, there is an exception to the safety of aspartame in this context. For those people, with a rare genetic disorder known as phenylketonuria, aspartame is not recommended.

Phenylketonuria occurs in roughly one out of every 15,000 people. Individuals with this disorder inherit one defective gene from each parent. They cannot process phenylalanine properly, and as a result, it accumulates to toxic levels that can result in mental retardation in children if the disorder is not diagnosed in a timely fashion. For this reason, many states require a blood test for phenylketonuria as part of newborn testing. While aspartame raises phenylalanine levels in people with phenylketonuria only slightly, it is still a concern because these individuals actually have to monitor their phenylalanine intake quite carefully.

While people who have phenylketonuria should not use aspartame, those who only have one phenylketonuria gene have no problem with it. Even those mothers who may unwittingly be carrying a fetus with phenylketonuria have nothing to fear. As long as they do not have the illness themselves, their bodies will process aspartame properly and thereby keep phenylalanine levels normal.

Methanol is the third and final metabolite of aspartame. Toxic in large doses, methanol is a normal by-product of digestion. The amount of methanol produced from a single can of artificially sweetened soda is approximately the same as that from a banana and less than that from an equal volume of several types of fruit juices. Even a dose of aspartame equivalent to sixty cans of soda at a single serving failed to change blood levels of methanol and its metabolites.

As can be seen, aspartame is broken down into naturally occurring products already found in our diets. No conceivable intake of aspartame can significantly alter the levels of these breakdown products found in our bloodstream. Short of suffocating in a boxcar of artificial sweetener, aspartame is as close as anything else in our diet to being "perfectly safe" for children, adults, and pregnant women.

What about the notion that Nutrasweet (aspartame) is safer than sugar? As can be seen from the preceding discussion, no conceivable dose (even excessive in the eyes of scientists) was able to significantly alter body chemistry even at the time of consumption. Does sugar meet this standard?

Sugar, a "natural" component of our diet, provides four calories for every gram—four times the number of calories for an equal weight of protein. As a relatively high-calorie food, sugar consumption is directly related to weight. The fact that obesity has been linked to heart disease, cancer, and physical injuries is well established and widely known. Of course, a separate issue is the close association between sugar consumption and dental decay. No such bad consequences have been ascribed to Nutrasweet usage. While sugar clearly poses health threats to the general population, does it pose any special threats to pregnant women?

Pregnant women are not immune to tooth decay and the problems of obesity. While these tend to have longer term consequences, excessive weight gain also causes an immediate health threat to pregnant women. This occurs in the form of gestational diabetes and an increased risk of cesarean section.

Perhaps one to two percent of pregnant women will develop gestational diabetes. Typically occurring in the third trimester of pregnancy, this malady results when the body cannot adequately control sugar (glucose) levels in the bloodstream. As a result, the average blood level of sugar rises and the fetus tends to become larger than he or she might otherwise be. Also, the risk of stillbirth rises for gestational diabetics. Both of these undesirable outcomes tend to be minimized if gestational diabetes is diagnosed and treated. Nonetheless, no one would wish to develop diabetes during pregnancy regardless of medical care. Prepregnancy obesity has been linked to an increased risk of gestational diabetes. To the extent that sugar intake is related to weight, excess sugar intake can increase the risk for gestational diabetes and thereby fetal injury. Also, as noted above, extra weight gain clearly increases the risk of cesarean section. Rather than worry about Nutrasweet, expectant mothers should strive to start pregnancy at a good weight and avoid gaining extra pounds beyond what their doctor recommends.

As can be seen, Nutrasweet, an artificial sweetener, is safer than sugar, a "natural" dietary component. While Nutrasweet is not known or suspected to cause any type of ill effect as a dietary supplement, excessive sugar intake that results in obesity has been linked to a wide variety of bad outcomes. These dangers apply to the general population with additional risks of gestational diabetes and cesarean birth for pregnant women.

One of the reasons that this book came into being is because I have seen so many patients following the advice of their friends and others who have not been well informed. Although it may seem to be "common sense" for expectant mothers to discard the artificially sweetened soft drinks and substitute regular soda or fruit juices, it is dead wrong for anyone who is having trouble with excess weight gain. Even though most of my patients are well versed on the dangers of obesity, many of them seem are surprised to hear that sugar is not particularly "safe."

Myth #16:
Prenatal vitamins are very important diet supplements.

The average American consumer seems to have an overpowering belief in the potent health-restoring powers of vitamins. Such misplaced faith is hard to shake and stems from both a kernel of truth and the marketing efforts of the health food and vitamin industry.

A vitamin is defined as "One of a group of organic substances, present in minute amounts in natural foodstuffs, which are essential to normal metabolism and lack of which in the diet causes deficiency diseases." It was a breakthrough in medical science to realize that vitamin deficiency caused diseases. For instance, a lack of vitamin D in the diet results in rickets, often recognized by abnormal bone formation in children. An absence of dietary vitamin C causes scurvy, a disease that causes teeth to fall out and wounds to heal slowly.

If an absence of vitamins causes disease, does an excess bring about health? Obviously those who sell vitamins would like you to believe that this is so, and it seems logical. However, it simply has not been proven to be the case. For instance, there is no consensus that excess vitamin C helps prevent colds despite widespread belief that it does.

What about vitamins for the pregnant woman? It is worth emphasizing that vitamins are required only in minute amounts for normal bodily function. Any dietary intake that results in weight gain during pregnancy, particularly in the United States where many foods are fortified with vitamins, is likely to contain the appropriate amounts of vitamins. In fact, to quote directly from one obstetrics text, "The increased requirements for vitamins during pregnancy in practically all circumstances can be supplied by any general diet that provides adequate amounts of calories and protein." Another text states, "Prenatal vitamin-mineral supplements are widely prescribed and can provide a false sense of security about a woman's diet. After examining all of the available evidence regarding the safety issues and justification for vitamin and mineral supplementation during pregnancy, the Institute of Medicine has concluded that routine supplementation of any nutrient, excepting iron, is unwarranted."

In contrast to the lack of need for vitamin supplements, there are concerns about those who take vitamins to excess. Megadose vitamins (defined here as an intake of ten times or more of the recommended daily allowance) have been found to cause birth defects in animals. As a result, there is some concern about excessive doses of these nutrients taken by pregnant women.

There are two small exceptions to the idea that vitamin supplements provide no benefit to the properly nourished expectant woman. Iron, a mineral required in increased amounts for the production of fetal red blood cells, is so often deficient in the maternal diet that routine supplementation is frequently recommended. However, it is worth pointing out that without iron supplementation, the fetus invariable takes the needed iron from maternal stores. As a result, fetuses are almost never deficient—rather the mothers become low in iron. This is usually not a major problem as the expectant mother only becomes mildly anemic (lower in red blood cells). This pregnancy anemia is rarely severe enough to cause symptoms such as fatigue. Many people who are fatigued are quick to blame their symptoms on lack of iron and anemia even when their blood counts and iron stores are perfectly normal.

Folic acid is another exception to the general rule that pregnant women seldom, if ever, need to supplement their diet with vitamin pills. There is some recent evidence that supplementing the diet with folic acid prior to conception may reduce the risk of neural tube defects—a birth defect in which the spinal cord is not formed properly. As a result, the Centers for Disease Control recommend that all women anticipating conception take folic acid supplementation (folate) in the amount of 400 micrograms (or 0.4 milligrams) daily.

There is a bottom line to this discussion. Many women have the mistaken notion that vitamins can correct a poor diet to the point that their nutritional status becomes satisfactory for pregnancy. In reality, the exact opposite is true. A healthy diet makes vitamin supplementation unnecessary. These medicinal supplements cannot provide the calories and protein that every developing fetus so badly needs.

MYTH #17:
Pregnant women should not take medicine.

As with many myths, this one contains a kernel of truth. A very few medications are well known to cause birth defects in fetuses when taken during pregnancy. However, many medicines, including many of those required for the health of the mother, are not only safe for the fetus but actually beneficial to the extent that they improve maternal well-being.

There are several issues in considering the safety of medication. As a general rule, it is thought that the developing baby is most sensitive to the development of birth defects from environmental factors in the first trimester, the time of organ development. There is a major exception to this principal: during the first week or so after conception, the fetus seems to be relatively protected. Fortunately, this is the time before the first missed menstrual period—in other words, before a woman realizes that she may be pregnant. It is further theorized that at this time there are so few cells in the new conceptus that damage to any one of them would be critical, resulting in very early miscarriage rather than the birth at term of a damaged baby.

Fetal deformity is not the only concern when advising pregnant women on medication. Some drugs can interfere with metabolism in the newborn and thus are not typically used in the last few weeks of pregnancy. For instance, the use of sulfa antibiotics can predispose some newborns to jaundice when used immediately preceding birth.

In my interaction with other obstetricians as well as doctors in other specialties, I have found that their interest in and knowledge of the subject of teratogenicity (environmental causes of birth defects) varies considerably. Perhaps this is the cause of excessive caution in treating patients. Teratogenicity is a well-established scientific discipline, and answers not available to the practicing physician years ago are available today, literally at his or her fingertips. As an example, most obstetricians can get access to computerized data bases that are continuously updated with information on teratogenicity of various substances. If the drug in question is important to maintain good health, the pregnant woman should discuss it with her doctor.

With these considerations in mind, it is worth noting that of the several thousand medications available, only 30 or so are known to be teratogens (a cause of birth defects). Certainly this fact is not cited to encourage pregnant women to take medication with no thought for the developing child. Rather, this discussion is meant to provide balance. Sadly, many mothers are frightened out of taking medication that is necessary for them, which may be even beneficial to the fetus, or at least pose no danger. Thyroid hormone supplementation and most asthma medications come to mind as examples of necessary medication for maternal health that are appropriate to take in pregnancy.

MYTH #18:
It is okay for a pregnant woman to have an occasional drink of alcohol.

Of all the substances normally in our diet, only one readily comes to mind as a proven teratogen (a cause of birth defects)— alcohol. Alcohol consumption is clearly one of the most important environmental causes of mental retardation.

Fetal alcohol syndrome was first identified in 1973. Characterized by mental retardation, abnormal facial appearance, and behavioral disturbances, it is seen in the babies of up to 40 percent of women who are alcoholics. Other problems such as heart defects and brain abnormalities are also common. The alcohol consumption needed for fetal alcohol syndrome is approximately six drinks per day. In this context, a drink is defined as one beer, one glass of wine, or one mixed drink.

Less alcohol consumption is associated with a less severe abnormal outcome—fetal alcohol effects. These children are afflicted by mild mental deficiency, subtle behavioral abnormalities, and more mild anatomical abnormalities. These problems can be brought on by consumption of two to four drinks of alcohol daily.

"Binge" drinking, in which total consumption of alcohol is less but is in concentrated in bursts, is also suspected of posing grave dangers to the fetus. In monkeys, a single dose of eight drinks once during pregnancy has been shown to result in an increased miscarriage rate, facial abnormalities, and behavioral disturbances in the offspring.

In view of this data, what is a safe dose of alcohol consumption? NONE! As a practical matter, obstetricians do not expect deformed babies if a mother inadvertently has a few drinks before she realizes that she is pregnant. However, it is worth noting that alcohol is one of the few substances in our environment, whether it be in our diet, workplace, or medicine cabinet, that is absolutely proven to cause fetal injury. No safe minimum dose has been established. To put it as clearly as possible, "no alcohol" means no champagne on New Year's Eve, no social drinking, and no medication (such as some cold medicines) with significant alcohol content.

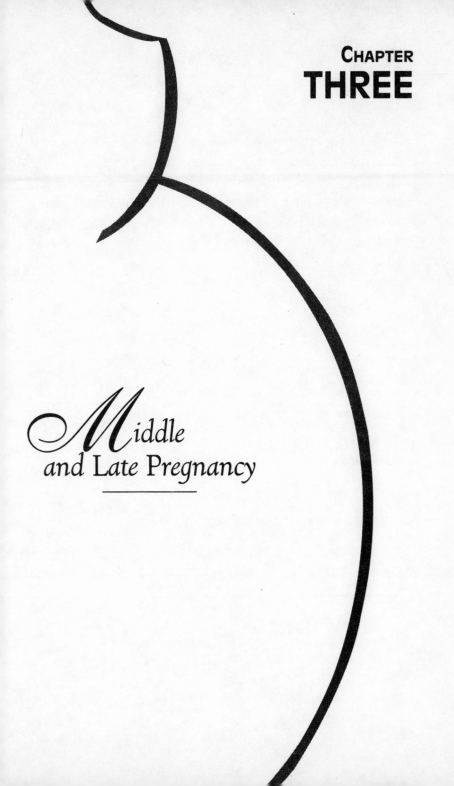

*M*iddle
and Late Pregnancy

Prenatal Testing

Since the AFP test has a high false positive rate, it should be refused.

This subject is so complex that in a face-to-face discussion between patient and doctor, it is my guess that most patients will accept their doctor's guidance without really understanding the issues. As with many myths, it contains a kernel of truth; this along with its complexity makes it more difficult to debunk.

"AFP" stands for alpha-fetoprotein. This is a protein produced by embryonic tissues. The molecule enters the maternal bloodstream and can be measured simply by taking a sample of the pregnant woman's blood. Unfortunately, the amount of the protein in the bloodstream does not always correspond to a specific level in the amniotic fluid. Fetuses with birth defects in which nerve tissue is open to the outside usually have elevated levels of AFP in both the amniotic fluid and the maternal blood stream. Also known as neural tube defects (NTDs), the most common type is spina bifida in which the spinal cord has no covering and is in direct contact with the outside. These babies are typically paralyzed below the waist and incontinent.

Since the introduction of the AFP test, it has become evident that abnormally low levels of AFP are associated with an increased rate of Down's syndrome. With Down's syndrome, the fetus has three number 21 chromosomes instead of the usual two and is often stillborn or severely retarded. Unlike for NTDs, the risk of such chromosome errors increases with maternal age.

To return to the issues raised by the above myth, what is a "false positive test result"? Even more to the point, what is a "high rate"? Medical tests are generally evaluated by their sensitivity and specificity. A sensitive test is one that will detect the presence of disease if present. Specificity is the idea that a test will be abnormal only in the presence of disease. As a rule, test results can be classified with the following method:

	Positive Test Results	
	Abnormal (positive) Result	Normal (negative) Result
Patient really has disease	True Positive	False Negative
Patient does not really have disease	False Positive	True Negative

Obviously, doctors and patients want to use tests that always have true positives and true negatives. What good is the test if it misses disease or diagnoses illness in a healthy person? Unfortunately, we do not live in utopia and most medical tests are not 100 percent sensitive and 100 percent specific.

For example, the news media recently caused a storm of attention to focus on the "inaccuracy" of pap smears. The journalists were not able to distinguish between two issues—the inherent (and well-known) limitations of the test accuracy and the presence of poorly run labs. For instance, it is medical dogma that in the best labs, a pap may miss an occasional cancer (the test is not 100 percent sensitive). Conversely, the test will occasionally show an abnormality in a woman with a perfectly normal cervix (the test is not 100 percent specific). Does this less-than-perfect test have value? Of course! Since its introduction several decades ago, the death rate from cervical cancer has dropped remarkably. It would drop even further if women were more conscientious about getting them annually. Yet the news media did have a story: there are a few corrupt or careless labs. By confusing the issues, the media convinced many people that corrupt labs were commonplace, and as a result, the pap smear test has little value. So it is with the AFP test. The fact that the test is imperfect does not mean that has no value.

To improve the accuracy of the AFP test, two other molecules are commonly measured at the same time, HCG (human chorionic gonadotropin) and estriol. The measurement of these additional molecules seems to improve the accuracy of the AFP test though there is no national consensus on test methodology. The numbers cited below refer to the plain AFP test although the general principles also apply to the more recent combination tests.

There are roughly one to two babies per 1,000 born in the United States with some type of neural tube defect. The rate of Down's syndrome varies according to maternal age but for a 25 year-old the risk is about one to two per 1,000; for that of a 35-year-old the risk is three to four per 1,000. As can be seen, for every thousand women tested, one or two will be carrying a child with an NTD and approximately the same number will be carrying a baby with Down's syndrome.

What happens with the AFP test? Of 1,000 women, 25 to 50 will have a high AFP value and 40 to 50 will have a low value. Phrased differently, up to 10 percent of the population will have an abnormal test result. For those 50 women with a high level, a repeat level will be abnormal again in 30 to 40 women. When these women have a follow-up ultrasound, the abnormal result will be explained for almost half of the cases (i.e., wrong gestational age, twins, etc.). The medical literature suggests that this will leave 17 to 18 women per thousand with an unexplained high result. Amniocentesis is recommended for this group. Of these women, only one or two fetuses will be found to have an NTD.

For a low level, the evaluation is slightly different. Suffice it to say that the low result will be unexplained in approximately 27 women. Of this group, only one woman on average after amniocentesis will actually be found to have a fetus with Down's syndrome.

Is this a "high false positive rate"? I do not know. Phrased differently, of every 1,000 women who get the conventional AFP test, an amniocentesis will be recommended for roughly 45 women. In this group, only three fetuses on average will actually be abnormal. Forty-two women will have undergone an amniocentesis despite the fact that they had been carrying a normal baby all along.

Perhaps some perspective is in order. Down's syndrome and NTDs are devastating problems. Life span is often greatly shortened and these individuals have a substantially reduced quality of life. The strain on the parents is enormous. For this reason, a great deal of effort seems warranted to identify these pregnancies. For example, the traditional recommendation for amniocentesis for mothers age 35 and over is derived from the fact that the overall rate of chromosome errors for 35 years olds is roughly one in 170. With an amniocentesis miscarriage rate of one in 200, age 35 is the first year in which the chance of *finding* a problem exceeds the risk of *causing* a problem. It is common practice across the country to recommend an amniocentesis to women who will be 35 and over at the time of their due date. In my experience, most patients readily accept this advice.

With this perspective, the AFP test doesn't seem like such a bad deal—45 amnios to find three babies with a problem. In comparison, for 170 mothers age 35 at the time of delivery, 169 of them will have amnios for fetuses with normal chromosomes while only one will have a detected problem. As can be seen, the AFP test (like most medical tests) does have limitations in accuracy and can scare mothers who will ultimately be found to have normal pregnancies. However, abnormal test results can generally be established as true or false through amniocentesis. The birth defects in question are serious enough for most people so that the search is worth the effort.

On a personal note, all obstetricians loathe calling patients with abnormal AFP results. We know that most of these pregnancies are normal. The typical response is sobbing after our first two sentences, "I'm calling about your AFP test. There was a slight problem with it." A certain small percentage of patients actually "kill the messenger" and leave the practice when we call with this news. Understandably, some doctors denigrate the test and encourage patients to refuse it. As much as my partners and I dislike making these calls, the test seems worthwhile despite the worry it can cause.

MYTH #20:
Mothers opposed to abortion for birth defects should get genetic testing anyway because it can better prepare them for a problem.

I am distressed by this argument as I find it profoundly misleading. In general, I suggest that knowing that there is a serious problem with the fetus about which nothing can be done will make parental suffering *much worse*. It is a great deal like knowing the date of your death well in advance. As a rule, there is little (i.e., nothing) that can be done for the fetus while it is still in the womb. Also, the precise nature of the problem is often difficult to determine before birth. For those parents who would never terminate a pregnancy under any circumstances, genetic testing is probably a bad idea for most.

It should be noted that this is my view and not a "fact" per se. I know that many other doctors disagree with me on this point. Yet this disagreement comes from the observation common to all of us that even the most vigorous abortion opponent will often change positions when confronted with a severely abnormal fetus. Nonetheless, I think that a patient's philosophical viewpoint should be respected. In practice, little can be done for severe defects before birth. I suspect that the physician's argument for genetic testing in those opposed to abortion is a sort of a smoke screen for the belief that the patient's position will change when actually faced with a difficult situation.

As an aside, the doctors in my practice are anxious to respect religious and philosophical beliefs. Yet when we try to explain genetic tests such as the AFP test to our patients, the room for miscommunication is great. When we first tried to explain that those opposed to abortion should not get the test, an occasional patient would misunderstand and somehow think that we were recommending an abortion for them. As a result, we now simply emphasize that the test is optional. However, if we already know someone would never abort (such as many of the divinity students in our care), we advise them against the test.

MYTH #21:

An abnormal screening test for diabetes strongly suggests that the patient has diabetes.

Diabetes is an illness in which the body fails to regulate sugar (glucose) levels in the bloodstream properly. The hormone insulin is a protein produced by the pancreas and is chiefly responsible for driving glucose out of the bloodstream and into cells. If glucose levels are too high, longterm damage to bodily organs can occur. With very excessive levels, patients can become quite sick in the short term. During pregnancy, the placenta produces a hormone, Human Placental Lactogen (HPL), that partially blocks the action of insulin. As a result, women who can produce enough insulin in the nonpregnant state occasionally develop a relative insulin deficiency at the end of pregnancy when HPL is produced in large amounts. Gestational diabetes can cause a modest increase in the rate of pregnancy complications.

Approximately one to two percent of the pregnant population will develop gestational diabetes in the third trimester. The screening test most commonly done for this problem is the one-hour glucose test. Patients are given a 50-gram glucose drink, and then their blood is drawn an hour later. Glucose levels above 140 milligrams/deciliter are considered abnormal. At this point, a three-hour glucose tolerance test is prescribed. In this test, a fasting glucose level is obtained, followed by levels at one, two, and three hours after a 100-gram glucose drink. If any two of the four levels on this second test are abnormal, the patient has gestational diabetes. In most cases, the initial treatment is a modified diet.

As with the discussion about the AFP test, the issues here are the sensitivity and specificity of the one-hour glucose test. While the one-hour screen will detect most women who actually have diabetes, most of those with an abnormal one-hour screen result will not have the disease. As noted above, one to two women out of every 100 will actually have gestational diabetes. About 15 out of 100 will have an abnormal one-hour test. Saying it another way, of the 15 women with the abnormal screen, only one or two will subsequently have an abnormal three-hour screen. This corresponds to an 87 percent chance (13/15) that those who flunk the one-hour test will pass the three-hour test.

Why do so many normal people have a high one-hour test? There are two reasons. First, there is a considerable overlap in the glucose levels between patients with and without gestational diabetes. The cut-off glucose level has to be set low enough so that those few people who are diabetic will be identified. Second, sugar levels do vary even in normal patients and the level can be momentarily high due to chance. If the one-hour test is so imprecise, why bother with it? While it is true that most people with an abnormal glucose screen actually do not have diabetes, 85% of the population have a normal test result. This majority are spared the inconvenience of a the three-hour test. Ultimately, the medical profession had to make a recommendation for one of two choices given the desire to detect those few women with gestational diabetes. Screen everyone with a one-hour test and accept some false positives or give everyone the three-hour test and eliminate false positives altogether. In the scheme currently described, 85 women out of every hundred undergo a simple one hour-test while the remaining 15 have to get tested twice. Even so, there remains controversy within our specialty as to whether everyone should be screened or whether the screen should be limited to patients with established risk factors.

Activity

MYTH #22:
Pregnant women should use care not to sleep on their backs.

This was a particularly vexing issue to deal with since obstetrical texts do not comment on it despite the fact that it seems to be a widespread belief among the general population. In reviewing the medical literature, a variety of observations can be collected to suggest that this advice is either wrong or unnecessary.

A condition called "supine hypotensive syndrome" is well known among maternity personnel. In late pregnancy, a substantial number of women are prone to experience a drop in blood pressure with the concomitant symptoms of dizziness and light-headedness. If positioned flat on their back during anesthesia, the blood pressure can drop low enough on occasion to become a threat to the health of mother and baby. Does this have any relevance for pregnant women not undergoing anesthesia or surgery at the moment? Probably not much.

In a review article of 100 published studies and reports in the medical literature, the authors made a variety of observations that are relevant to this issue. First, virtually all of the women predisposed to fainting while lying flat on their back developed symptoms that made them uncomfortable in this position. They avoided this posture so effectively that they even shifted positions in sleep. Second, "the syndrome on its own has not been shown to have produced any maternal morbidity or mortality." That is, there does not seem to be a single case in the medical literature in which a mother or fetus suffered any injury whatsoever from the mother falling asleep on her back. Finally, sleeping on one's back does not seem to be very popular among pregnant women, symptoms or no symptoms. In another paper, only one pregnant woman out of 51 slept on her back in the third trimester.

In summary, the advice that makes the best sense is also so obvious that it barely needs stating: "Sleep in your most comfortable position." For those few pregnant women who are most comfortable sleeping on their back, the very fact that they are comfortable is good evidence that they are not jeopardizing their health or that of the fetus.

MYTH #23:
Pregnant women should not exercise.

There are a number of issues raised by this myth. Naturally many physical changes occur as the pregnancy progresses that will diminish a woman's capacity for vigorous exercise. Baseline oxygen consumption increases by 10–20 percent, resulting in an increased respiratory rate and cardiac output at rest. What's more, a substantial amount of the blood supply is diverted to the uterus (and developing fetus). As a result, there is decreased oxygen available for aerobic exercise and most pregnant women will fatigue earlier than they might otherwise, particularly in the third trimester. Another issue is the pregnant woman's ability to dissipate heat build-up during exercise as there are concerns about longterm exposure of the fetus to high core temperatures. Fortunately, pregnant women show a slower rise in internal body temperature than nonpregnant women and this theoretical concern has not been borne out in practice.

With these facts in mind, what exercise can a pregnant woman do? In essence she has no specific restrictions. Of course, common sense has a key role to play here. Pregnant women should not exercise so vigorously that they experience pain, exhaustion, or other symptoms of extreme fatigue such as dizziness. (These rules are probably appropriate for everyone, pregnant or not.) One unique restriction for pregnant women that seems well merited, however, is the suggestion that they do not exercise while lying flat on their back after the first trimester. (This restriction does not apply to sleeping on one's back.) In this position, the fetus rests on major blood vessels, making the body less able to accommodate increases in pulse and oxygen consumption.

Also, a special word of caution is in order in the third trimester for those upright activities that require balance or sudden changes in direction. With greater weight, a higher center of gravity, and possible increased laxity in the joints due to the hormones of pregnancy, it is typically more difficult to move rapidly. This may predispose one to falling and injury. Consequently, activities such as running and tennis should be undertaken with caution.

MYTH #24:
Stretching can choke the baby by kinking (or stretching) the umbilical cord.

While this is a common misconception, there is no specific discussion of it that I could find in the medical literature (probably because it would never occur to researchers to take this issue too seriously). From a certain common sense point of view, this idea would appear to have logic, although it is wrong for a variety of reasons.

The umbilical cord is actually cushioned by a fair amount of fat that protects the two arteries and one vein contained within. Rather than having the limpness of strands of cooked spaghetti, the cord has the tenseness of wire. It does not kink easily nor is it very compressible. Furthermore, the cord generally has excess length so that it permits a great deal of movement from the fetus without being placed under tension. Also, the fetus and umbilical cord are actually suspended in the amniotic fluid, which provides a great deal of cushioning from maternal movement and external pressure. Finally, fetuses can and do move all the time. This would naturally tend to reduce the possibility of any stretching or kinking. Given the cushioning of the umbilical cord, its physical resiliency, and its suspension in amniotic fluid, kinking or damage from maternal movement or stretching should be of no concern.

MYTH #25:
Lifting heavy objects can damage the baby.

Lifting itself poses no special problem for the fetus since it is the maternal skeletal muscles that are involved in the lifting effort. Of course, common sense should apply. Pregnant women should not lift more than they would when not pregnant, since this predisposes them to injury (pregnant or not). Pregnant women, particularly in the third trimester, are more prone to injury simply because they weigh more, their center of gravity is higher, and the hormones of pregnancy loosen the pelvic joints. So while fetal injury is not a concern, maternal injury from imprudent lifting is an issue. As an aside, heavy amounts of physical labor in an occupational setting may be linked to increased risk for preterm labor.

MYTH #26:

Pregnant women should not go horseback riding.

There is no medical literature that I could find for or against horseback riding during pregnancy. However, it appears safe to address the two obvious concerns with this activity. First, there is simply nothing to suggest that bouncing up and down in the saddle poses any unique threat to the fetus. As noted previously, normal pregnancies are very difficult indeed to shake loose. The second objection is more of a concern: falling off the horse. As the horse has some height and would usually be moving when the rider falls (or is thrown), it is easy to imagine significant injury occurring. While broken bones seem to be the most likely outcome, it may be possible to injure the soft organs including the uterus. However, the dictum against falling off horses clearly should not be applied only to pregnant women, but to all riders, male and female. Whether pregnant or not, riders should be knowledgeable about the dangers of falls. In this context, if a pregnant woman is a competent rider, it seems reasonable to permit horseback riding. She just has one more reason to be careful.

Environmental Dangers

MYTH #27:

Hot baths are dangerous for the fetus.

This myth has a variety of relatives including prohibitions on hot tubs, saunas, and showers as well. Its lineage can be traced to some very spotty data suggesting an increased risk of birth defects in mothers who are exposed to heat extremes (i.e., prolonged high fevers, etc.). Unfortunately, the data in this area is somewhat skimpy though some general conclusions can be drawn.

Assuming that prolonged, significant rises in temperature are undesirable, it is important to be precise. It is core temperature that is at issue. Such temperature is at the center of the body and is not skin temperature. Since mammals have a variety of systems for regulating core temperature in response to environmental changes, core temperatures simply do not change very quickly or drastically in most circumstances.

Another issue often overlooked is the fact that significant rises in core temperature can lead to significant discomfort and symptoms in the expectant mother herself. For this reason many hot tubs have posted warnings to limit bathing to a specified amount of time. In experiments cited in the medical literature, few people could tolerate staying in a hot tub or sauna that actually caused a significant rise in core temperature.

In considering the dangers of warm water, the three types of exposure should be distinguished. It is probably impossible to cause a significant change in core temperature with a hot shower. Even if the water is so hot that it actually scalds the skin, the small surface area and rapid evaporation of the water droplets eliminate hot showers as a method to raise core temperature. The other extreme, complete immersion in warm water up to the neck, is more of a concern since evaporation and other methods of heat radiation are neutralized. The effects of a tub baths, in which water is rarely more than a foot deep, resemble those of showers more than hot tubs. It is very unlikely that core temperature would change substantially since much of the body is still able to radiate heat into the surrounding air.

At the present, the consensus in the medical literature seems to limit hot tub and sauna exposure to 15 minutes. This is probably a good rule of thumb anyway, depending on the temperature of the devices, since large changes in core temperature can affect non-pregnant persons adversely. In contrast, sitting in a foot or so of hot water or taking a warm shower probably has no upper time limit of safety (other than local burns if the water is too hot).

MYTH #28:
Do not let children play in the sandbox for fear of toxoplasmosis.

Toxoplasmosis is a parasite whose most common relevant host is domestic cats. The disease is not typically spread from human to human but rather from cats to humans. An active case of toxo-plasmosis during pregnancy is not very common—it is estimated to occur only 1 in 1,000 pregnancies. For those with active infections, the parasite can cause injury to fetuses, including inflammations of the eyes and mental retardation. Congenital infection is more common among mothers who acquire toxoplasmosis in the third trimester, though first trimester infections tend to be more severe. At the present, the American College of Obstetricians and Gynecologists does not recommend routine screening.

The disease is normally acquired by inhaling or ingesting the toxoplasmosis eggs found in the feces of infected house cats. As a result, pregnant women should not change cat litter. In practice, cat owners may find it difficult to eliminate all chance of infection since the parasite's eggs easily become aerosolized and may remain infective for weeks. With regard to the above myth, toxo-plasmosis is not typically transmitted between humans so that in the extreme case of a child becoming infected, the risk to his/her mother is low. Also, playground sandboxes are by no means the same as kitty litter and simply do not pose a meaningful risk. Fortunately, toxoplasmosis remains a relatively rare threat for pregnant women.

MYTH #29:
Pregnant women should not perm their hair.

Though certainly not necessary for reasons of health, many pregnant women wish to continue to use permanent wave preparations. Current evidence suggests that it is safe and reasonable to do so. This two-step process is not known to use substances that cause birth defects in animals and no systemic toxicity is known or suspected. Adverse reactions are typically limited to local dermatitis of the scalp. Nonetheless, it seems prudent to wear gloves during the process and avoid leaving the solution in contact with the scalp for excessive periods of time.

Symptoms

MYTH #30:
Preeclampsia occurs in 20 percent of pregnancies.

This myth is one that I heard stated with some authority when my wife and I took Lamaze classes during our first pregnancy. (I did not correct the instructor.) While I do not think that anyone in class could have quoted this false statistic from memory, it definitely gives lay persons the impression that preeclampsia is more common than it really is.

Preeclampsia, also known as toxemia, is an illness unique to pregnant women. Characterized by high blood pressure, excessive loss of protein in the urine, and swelling, it is typically confined to the third trimester. The most commonly cited incidence rate is 5 percent (or one out of every twenty women). The statistics can vary greatly, depending on the population studied. It usually does not occur in subsequent pregnancies. Its cause is unknown, but it is invariably cured by delivery of the fetus.

MYTH #31:
A pregnant woman who has swelling probably has preeclampsia.

The reader will note that swelling is part of the definition of preeclampsia described earlier. While traditionally one of the three components used to diagnose this malady, swelling is now recognized to be so commonplace in pregnancy that there is controversy about the role swelling should play in diagnosing preeclampsia. In any case, it can be fairly stated that the majority of pregnant women have some sort of swelling by the end of pregnancy, while the majority clearly do not have this illness. While it may be true that the majority of women with preeclampsia have swelling, the converse clearly is not the case—the majority of women with swelling do *not* have preeclampsia.

How can a pregnant woman tell whether her swelling is normal or due to preeclampsia? In a word, she cannot. Swelling should be considered to be a usual part of pregnancy unless told otherwise by her physician. Preeclampsia is diagnosed by checking blood pressure and checking the urine for abnormal amounts of protein. The prenatal visits increase in frequency in the third trimester specifically to monitor for this complication. Swelling is so commonplace in late pregnancy that that in itself should be no cause for concern.

MYTH #32:

Headache is a symptom of high blood pressure.

This myth is not confined to pregnant women but is certainly quoted by some. High blood pressure does not cause people to *feel* sick. It does not cause recognizable symptoms. This is why longterm high blood pressure is often called "the silent killer." There is no "normal" blood pressure. As a general rule the lower the blood pressure is, the longer the life span. This terminology refers to the pressure at which the heart pumps blood through the blood vessels. It is typically described as two numbers. The top number (systolic) is peak pressure generated by the heart while actually contracting. The bottom number (diastolic) is the minimum pressure in the blood vessels between cardiac contractions. Just as pushing water through a garden hose with greater and greater force will cause the hose to wear out more quickly, so it is with high blood pressure and the blood vessels. Also, the pump (i.e., the heart) will fail sooner when working harder. The cause of high blood pressure is poorly understood.

As stated above, high blood pressure does not cause symptoms and certainly is not responsible for headache. There is a small exception (so rare that one wonders if it should even be mentioned). In those few patients with extremely elevated blood pressures (diastolic of 130 or so and greater), a headache can be a warning symptom of an impending stroke. These patients require immediate hospitalization in an intensive care unit so that their blood pressure can be quickly lowered. This is so uncommon that most gynecologists will not encounter a single case in their entire career. Internists, who deal more often with people who have longstanding hypertension, may encounter this on rare occasions.

MYTH #33:

Leg cramps are a symptom of blood clots.

Leg cramps are painful spasms from muscle contractions. Common to runners during the fatigue experienced after long races, they occur also more frequently in pregnant women. These leg cramps have nothing to do with blood clots. Indeed, deep-vein blood clots that are dangerous are fortunately quite rare, occurring in less than one out of every 1,000 pregnancies.

MYTH #34:

Leg cramps are caused by a lack of calcium.

While this is a popular and widespread myth, relatively little investigation on this subject has been noted in the medical literature. Contained within the few papers that deal with the subject are highly speculative and tentative suggestions that calcium may have a role to play in either the cause or treatment of leg cramps. Fortunately, at least one thorough study has been done, and it seems to be reasonably conclusive that calcium does not play a role in causing leg cramps.

This study consisted of 60 pregnant women with leg cramps who underwent treatment with either calcium or vitamin C. Neither the patients nor the doctors knew which substance was being administered (a double blind trial). Of interest was that the majority of participants from both groups experienced an improvement in symptoms (due to a placebo effect or spontaneous improvement). No group of patients in this study had any difference in calcium levels in the bloodstream. That is, those whose symptoms improved did not have different calcium levels than those who did not. Parenthetically, the patients taking calcium supplementation did not increase their calcium levels even though they were taking substantial doses.

This report should lay to rest the idea that leg cramps are caused by lack of calcium or that calcium supplements can treat them. While calcium supplements are not the answer, pregnant women with leg cramps need not lose hope—they typically improve periodically during the pregnancy as demonstrated by the fact that most of the patients in the above study improved whether they were taking calcium or not.

Preparing for and Predicting Labor

MYTH #35:
It is possible to predict a woman's labor pattern from knowing her mother's labor pattern.

Again, I seem to be on my own here with regard to the medical literature. This widely held idea simply has not been studied formally by researchers. However, it is easy to predict what science would find if this issue were investigated: there is no predictive value in knowing the labor history of a pregnant patient's mother.

Closer scrutiny of the issues surrounding labor length can be quite revealing. First, it is extremely well established that with the same woman, second and subsequent labors are generally quite different from the first. However, while second labors and beyond are typically (not always) shorter and easier than the first, they can vary greatly among the same woman. In other words, knowing a patient's prior labor history does not permit doctors to predict her future labors with great accuracy. As an extreme example of this, women who have undergone cesarean section for failure to progress in one pregnancy can actually deliver vaginally 80 percent of the time in the very next pregnancy!

Another issue is the weight and shape of the baby. While the relationship between these parameters and the course of labor is not well understood, mother and daughter are not likely to have babies of identical weight and shape. For one thing, the daughter has only 50 percent of her mother's genetic material—her bone structure and shape will clearly not be identical. The fetus itself, will have 50 percent of its genetic material from the father. Clearly there are numerous reasons to expect the daughter's labor experience to be unrelated to her mother's labor experience.

One final fact that should be noted to put this myth to rest is the considerable change that has taken place in obstetrical care over the last 30 years. For example, we now recommend 30-pound weight gains for the typical mother rather than the 15-pound weight gains commonly prescribed in the 1940s and 1950s. We do not give general anesthetics but we do give epidurals. Pitocin is now readily used and given via a computerized pump. We have internal pressure catheters that utilize a microchip to accurately measure uterine contractions in labors that are progressing slowly.

We cannot predict a patient's labor course from her mother's history because: 1) the labor experience is so highly variable from one pregnancy to the next in the same woman, 2) the patient and her mother never have identical anatomy, 3) the fetus has a completely different gene pool (and therefore weight and shape), and 4) obstetrical practice has changed significantly over the past three decades.

MYTH #36:

Braxton Hicks contractions are different than labor contractions.

I used to joke with my patients by asking them to guess the name of the two doctors who discovered "Braxton Hicks" contractions. The joke was on me since I subsequently learned that contractions before the onset of labor were first described in 1872 by *one person,* J. Braxton Hicks. While it was an important observation at the time, the designation of these prelabor contractions by a specific name has led to a lot of misunderstandings about both labor and contractions.

Labor is defined as regular contractions that result in steady cervical thinning and dilation. As such, the diagnosis of labor is made retrospectively: did the cervix change over time? Experienced labor and delivery personnel can often look at a patient and have some idea about how likely it is that she is dilating, but even we are fooled from time to time. Mothers in preterm labor can often have hours of regular mild contractions that do result in dilation and ultimately delivery. To make matters more confusing, many mothers have hours of regular contractions that do *not* result in dilation and then these contractions disappear.

Giving contractions a specific name is misleading in that it implies that somehow one type of contraction is inherently different than another type. Actually, this is not the case. As described above, some mothers with mild regular contractions can deliver while others with very painful contractions do not dilate and then the contractions stop.

The idea of a special type of contraction called a Braxton Hicks contraction no longer has any meaning. In fact, some authors in the medical literature have even made the astute observation that naming contractions before term "Braxton Hicks" and then calling them "normal" has caused some mothers to ignore the early symptoms of preterm labor. This idea should be discarded and replaced with a more pragmatic approach: "When should I call the doctor with contractions?"

The answer as to when the doctor should be called can be divided into two parts: before 36 weeks and after. The purpose of monitoring contractions more than four weeks before the due date is to be aware of the early symptoms of preterm labor so that should they occur, the labor can be interrupted and the pregnancy allowed to continue. To this end, anyone who has four or more contractions in an hour for two consecutive hours should notify her physician or caregiver. In most cases, the contractions will stop shortly and no special action will be required. Nonetheless, the doctor should be notified if they persist for two hours or more. Note that many women can have 10 or 20 contractions in a day, and this is not a concern. However, regular contractions that persist warrant medical advice.

Within four weeks of the due date, the issue is not so much prolonging the pregnancy but knowing when labor is beginning. Because many women notice an increase in the general frequency of contractions toward the end of pregnancy, this can be confusing. In the absence of other advice, first-time mothers should call their caregivers when their contractions are coming every five minutes for an hour. Second-time mothers (and third and fourth, etc.) should call earlier—when their contractions are every ten minutes for an hour. With these parameters, patients are reasonably likely to be starting to dilate when they call.

MYTH #37:

Braxton Hicks contractions help dilate the cervix.

From the discussion above, it can be seen that the concept of Braxton Hicks contractions has lost its meaning. Perhaps this question can be phrased a better way, "Do contractions before the onset of labor help dilate the cervix?" While the process of labor and cervical dilation is poorly understood, there is no evidence at the present time that these isolated contractions result in cervical change. Many women can experience literally hundreds of contractions over days and weeks with no discernable softening, thinning, or dilation of the cervix. It is this fact that makes it difficult for both doctor and patient to determine when labor begins. Ultimately, when there is a question, the only way to know what is happening is to actually check the cervix through examination.

MYTH #38:

Women are more likely to go into labor during a full moon.

This myth is often cited by labor nurses when maternity is busy during a full moon. Oddly enough, there is little reference by the medical staff to the same full moon when the labor and deliver suites are rather empty. Despite the fact that this "correlation" between labor and the full moon seems to be rather bizarre, medical literature, nevertheless, is not unanimous on this subject.

Two studies found no relationship between the lunar cycle and birth. The first, out of Denmark, examined 1,269 spontaneous labors over a two-year period. The second study evaluated 5,226 births over 37 lunar cycles and could find no link between labor onset and lunar status. In contrast, a French study, which used a very specialized statistical analysis of approximately six million births, was able to demonstrate a difference between the last week of the lunar month and the first week of the lunar month.

What can one conclude from these conflicting studies? Since the only study which could demonstrate a difference required six million births and compared two seven-day periods it seems fair to say that in small populations (i.e., of several thousand) any effect of the lunar cycle would be so small it would not be noticed. In fact, in two studies with smaller populations, it was not noticed. As a practical matter, it seems safe to conclude that the effect of the lunar cycle is so small (if it exists at all) that it does not have any meaning for individuals. Also, it is worth noting that the French study did not suggest an increased birth rate on the *day* of the full moon; rather that the rate increased during the seven days before hand in comparison with the seven days afterward.

MYTH #39:
Pregnant women are more likely to break their bag of waters during storms.

No doubt about it, this myth was derived from the meteorological observation that atmospheric pressure drops during thunderstorms. Unfortunately, this isolated truth neglected the fact that pressure within the body is always equal to pressure outside of the body. If this were not *always* true, we would burst or collapse regularly as the weather changed. Any drop in barometric pressure is matched by a corresponding drop in the pressure within the body.

The final doom for this myth is spelled out by a Danish study of 1,500 births over a two-year period. The investigators could find no relationship between rupture of membranes before the onset of labor and barometric pressure.

MYTH #40:
Doctors can predict who will need a cesarean by measuring the pelvis before labor.

Many patients who wind up with a cesarean section after a long labor are understandably frustrated. "Why couldn't they have figured out that I needed a cesarean before I want through all that labor?" The most common reason for cesarean section is cephalo-pelvic disproportion, or more simply stated, the fetus could not fit through the maternal pelvis. Unfortunately, even with present-day technology, it is impossible to predict who will get stuck and who will deliver.

The difficulty in making these predictions is rooted in several causes. First, determination of fetal size is notoriously inaccurate whether it is done either by physical exam or ultrasound. We simply cannot guess weights reliably. Second, even if the weight were known with certainty, the shape of fetuses with a given weight would vary widely. Third, accurate measurement of the bony structures in the maternal pelvis is so difficult that even X-ray measurements have largely been discredited. Finally, the dimension of both the fetus and the maternal pelvis are known to change some during labors. As can be seen, predicting the ease with which one complex three-dimensional structure will fit through another when both actually change their dimensions during the process is no trivial undertaking. Predicting which fetuses will deliver vaginally simply cannot be done reliably. There is simply no way to tell with certainty without going through the trial-and-error test of labor itself.

MYTH #41:

The doctor can predict when labor will start
by means of a cervical examination near the end of pregnancy.

Patients often ask during the pelvic exam at the end of pregnancy, "Have you changed my due date?" It is worth emphasizing that the due date and the actual arrival of the baby are two completely different (if not related) things. The due date is assigned 280 days after the first day of the last menstrual period. As such, it is intended to serve as the midpoint of the four-week time period when delivery is most likely to occur. The due date is never changed on the basis of information acquired in the third trimester such as cervical dilation or fetal size. The doctor may or may not make a statement predicting delivery on the basis of cervical exams, but he or she is not thereby changing the due date.

Does the state of the cervix provide additional information about when labor will start? Yes and no. It appears that in large populations, differences in cervical dilation are weakly associated with variations in the time to onset of labor. As a practical matter, the relationship is too weak to have much predictive accuracy when it comes to specific individuals.

The evidence that the status of the cervix is related to subsequent onset of delivery comes from two places. The first, the so-called Bishop score, is used to predict the success of induction of labor should delivery be necessary. The softer, more effaced, and more dilated the cervix, the more likely induction of labor will succeed. The second line of evidence suggesting that cervical dilation has some bearing on the time course to delivery is the fact that excessive dilation prematurely is linked in some cases to preterm labor. However, this relationship is a weak one since three-fourths of the women in one study who were dilated to two or three centimeters at 30 weeks gestation did not deliver until at least eight weeks later!

While the available information provides indirect evidence that there is a relationship between cervical dilation and the time course to delivery, the issue has never been examined with regard to when labor will start. From my own observations and what is described in the literature, it is clear that the relationship is a weak one. By this I mean that one could probably safely speculate that the average time to delivery for 1,000 first-time mothers dilated to two centimeters 14 days before their due date will be less than a similar group of patients who are not dilated at all. However, as the averages between the two groups probably would not be different by more than a few days and there would be considerable overlap, the information would have little predictive value for a specific individual. So while the idea that the doctor can predict the time of delivery from cervical exams has a small amount of validity, the concept in practice is much more misleading than helpful.

Myth #42:
First-time mothers tend to deliver late and second-time mothers tend to deliver early (or vice versa).

The due date is the average duration of the gestation from the first day of the last menstrual period (not ovulation or the time of conception). Studies of thousands of women consistently determine this interval to be 280 days with 90 to 95 percent of deliveries occurring within the time interval extending from 14 days or so before the due date to 14 days after the due date. Interestingly enough, a recent study from Sweden, in which over

400,000 pregnancies were evaluated, found that the average gestational length for women on their second or subsequent pregnancies was 12 to 24 hours less than that for first-time mothers.
However, both groups were equally likely to deliver both before
and after their average gestational length. Only about 4 percent of
the population actually delivered on the due date. The idea that the
due date represents the midpoint of the expected time of delivery
remains valid no matter how many times a woman has delivered
before.

MYTH #43:
I should donate blood before delivery.

Except possibly in those few circumstances in which a patient is
scheduled far in advance for a cesarean delivery on a specific day,
obstetricians do not generally recommend auto-donation. The
overall probability of requiring blood during childbirth is rather
low—on the order of 1 percent. Phrased differently, 99% of those
donating blood would have the blood wasted. (Blood banks generally do not transfer auto-donations to others.) Among those who
require blood, it is very difficult to predict the need with certainty
in advance. In one study, only four of 251 patients with risk factors
for blood loss ultimately needed blood. Also, if the donation
occurred immediately before delivery, it might actually increase
the need for blood. Finally, the vast majority of patients who are
transfused get more than one pint of blood. Even auto-donation
cannot significantly reduce the chance of getting at least a partial
transfusion with someone else's blood.

While the medical literature is relatively quiet on the subject of
auto-donation in anticipation of delivery, the one study that I could

find was openly skeptical. In general, it seems to be a fair amount of effort for little, if any, benefit.

Myth #44:
My family should donate blood for me before delivery.

This idea has to be debunked in two parts. As cited above, the actual risk of a transfusion is rather low—less than 1 percent. However, a much more important issue is the safety of so-called designated donor blood versus anonymous donor blood. The blood bank industry has long been skeptical of the practice of patients soliciting relatives and friends for blood—and with good reason. The concern is that when people are solicited to give blood by others whom they know, they may be more prone to overlook risk factors for infection that might otherwise give them pause. For instance, a husband who has slept with a prostitute is not likely to bring this up to his wife when she asks him to donate. In contrast, anonymous volunteer donors (who do not get paid) are not under any compulsion to donate blood and are freer to decline to donate if they discover that they may have risk factors through the blood bank screening process.

Other, technical issues are worth mentioning with regard to designated donor blood. First, the blood has to be compatible. (Just because it is a family member does not mean that the person has the same blood type.) Also, the blood has to be screened for disease just as is any other blood. This typically takes a few days so that in practice, designated donor blood cannot be obtained in time for true emergencies (the only type in which obstetricians are prone to transfuse).

Thus far, there have been few studies directly comparing the safety of designated donors versus anonymous donor blood. Nonetheless, one such paper in the German literature actually suggested that the infectious disease rate might be higher in the designated donor group. (The data was complicated by the fact that a specific immigrant group was more prone to have designated donors so the groups were not strictly comparable.) Nonetheless, this should serve as a caution to those inclined to have their families donate.

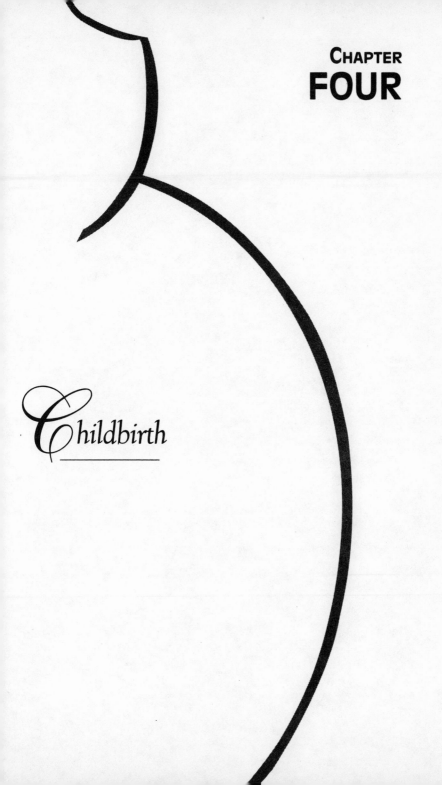

*C*hildbirth

The Amniotic Membranes

MYTH #45:
A "dry" birth is dangerous.

The "dry" birth in this myth simply refers to giving birth after the bag of waters has ruptured. While the myth expresses a natural concern for the baby if the bag containing the fluid breaks before the onset of labor, the fear of giving birth after this occurs is largely misplaced. Modern medical practice has been able to deal with this circumstance quite effectively. Known to obstetricians as premature rupture of membranes, this situation occurs about 10 percent of the time in full-term pregnancies. In most women this event typically causes labor to start within 24 hours.

As long as the membranes rupture at full term (within 14 days of the due date), the complication rate is low. While there is an increasing chance of infection after the membranes rupture, as a rule this risk rises only very slowly as time passes. The infection, chorioamnionitis, tends to be easily treated in both mother and baby, although there are exceptions. As for the lack of fluid to cushion the baby and the umbilical cord, this is not usually a concern for full term fetuses. Since problems can occasionally arise, women should notify their caregivers if there is a question about whether the membranes have broken. While not typically danger-ous, ruptured membranes require prompt examination and moni-toring by the medical staff.

MYTH #46:

A woman who had ruptured her bag of waters before the onset of labor in a previous labor is likely to do so in subsequent births.

Premature rupture of membranes (PROM) before term is known to increase a woman's risk of this complication occurring in a sub-sequent pregnancy. As noted above, PROM at term occurs in about 10 percent of the population; before term, it occurs one to two percent of the time. Preterm PROM has been studied more intensely than those cases at term. Women who have experienced preterm PROM are known to be at increased risk for a recurrence in subsequent pregnancies (in comparison to those who have not had preterm PROM). However, I was able to find at least one paper that specifically evaluated the risk of PROM at term if the patient had a history of PROM. This report found that mothers with such a history were approximately twice as likely to experi-ence this again in comparison with those who had not ruptured membranes before labor in a previous pregnancy.

The key issue here is that while those who experience PROM at term may be more likely to experience this event in subsequent pregnancies, the degree of risk is limited. Assuming that a woman who experienced PROM at term was twice as likely to have the same event on the next pregnancy, she would only have a 20 per-cent chance of having the bag of waters break before the onset of labor. Phrased another way, there would be an 80 percent chance that this would *not* happen. Also note that the risk of PROM is not known to be related to maternal age or number of prior pregnancies.

Pain Relief in Labor

MYTH #47:
Narcotic pain relief during labor is
inherently dangerous and should be avoided.

Narcotics like morphine are commonly used to relieve pain during labor (as well as after surgery). What are the dangers of this medication in laboring women? It should be said before reviewing the dangers, that such pain-relief medication is widely viewed by physicians as providing often much needed relief and its benefits far outweigh any risks from the medication itself.

In general, the chief danger is that the medication will suppress breathing. Narcotics in large doses are fatal because they shut down the brain's respiratory center and the patient will ultimately stop breathing. Fortunately, the difference between a fatal dose and that needed for relief of pain is sufficiently wide so that I cannot recall a single case of maternal respiratory depression requiring medical treatment among the thousands of laboring patients that I have observed.

However, medication given to laboring patients does make its way to the baby. For this reason, many obstetricians try not to administer such pain medications shortly before birth since they can cause decreased respiration in newborns. As noted above, in practice this is rarely a problem. Maternity staffs are also trained to assist newborns who do not breathe well on their own. Finally, for either mother or baby, there is a medication that can reverse the effects of narcotics within seconds should it be necessary. As a result, the risk of a substantial health danger from narcotic medication in labor and delivery is negligible.

Myth #48:

A common complication of epidural anesthesia is paralysis.

While epidural and spinal anesthetics can result in some complications, in general, the risk of serious injury or death from these procedures is exceedingly low. Of course, lay people imagine that paralysis is a major concern since in these procedures a needle is placed close to the spinal nerves. In two separate series of more than 10,000 patients receiving spinal anesthesia, not a single case of major neurologic injury was reported. For epidural anesthesia, the incidence of paralysis has been reported at the rate of two per 10,000 cases. For perspective, the death rate from auto accidents has been estimated at one per 6,000 people for only one year of driving. (The rate of major injury including paralysis is higher.)

Myth #49:

There is a substantial difference among
specific narcotics commonly prescribed in labor and delivery.

My patients will often state, "I have been told to be sure to ask you what type of medication you use in labor and delivery." When I reply "Stadol and Fentanyl," I am frequently greeted with blank stares. The simple truth is that all narcotics share common features. They cause respiratory depression and change (i.e., diminish) the perception of pain. They also have the same side effects to some extent: sedation and nausea. While manufacturers of one drug may claim fewer side effects than others, in practice any of the narcotics can have adverse effects. For maternity staffs, the important differences are in the areas of dosage, route of administration, time of onset, and duration of effect. Of course, if a patient remembers that previously she had been violently nauseated by a specific drug, we will try to use a different one. However, in many cases, the very same drug could be administered a second time with less adverse effects since the patient's basic condition is different from one episode of pain to the next.

MYTH #50:
Epidural anesthesia is safer than an injection of a narcotic.

This is another myth arising from the generally well-meaning instructors of childbirth classes. The statement that "epidural anesthesia is safer than an injection of narcotic" is incorrect, and in fact, the reverse is actually true. Moreover, the implication is that the narcotic injection should be avoided. While both methods of pain relief are so safe that rational people can request either one electively during labor, the risks of an epidural given to the mother and adversely affecting the fetus are clearly greater than with an injection of narcotic. As a result, the mechanics for administering these pain modalities are completely different. Epidurals are typically administered by anesthesiologists only after an intravenous line has been established to facilitate the rapid administration of fluids and medications if necessary. The patient is also connected to a continuous heart-rate monitor, and in my hospital (at the present time), an obstetrician has to be immediately available if the need should arise. In contrast, narcotic injections are typically given by labor nurses without an intravenous line and without the requirement of doctors in the immediate vicinity.

Labor

Myth #51:
Physical conditioning can have a significant impact on the course of labor.

Certainly it is reasonable to maintain physical conditioning during pregnancy and to continue to exercise. Regular exercise has been shown to reduce disease and injury and improve one's general sense of well-being. Unfortunately, all of this probably has little effect on the initiation, duration, or pain of labor.

During the first stage of labor, cervical dilation and descent of the fetus are mediated by the contractions of the uterus. This is made of smooth muscle over which there is no conscious control. There is no exercise or preparation known to affect the uterus in any way.

The second stage of labor, during which the cervix is completely dilated, is more complicated. During this part of labor, there is much that the mother can do to hasten delivery. This entails "pushing," in which the patient holds her breath and bears down. This serves to increase abdominal pressure and it certainly does appear that maternal efforts can have some impact on the length of this portion of labor. Nevertheless, it is impossible (and not even advisable) to practice this expulsive effort before it is actually needed.

Does a woman who does vigorous exercise to strengthen her abdominal muscles have an advantage over one who does not?

The answer is not known, though several observations are in order. First, exercising while lying flat on one's back is generally not recommended during the later part of pregnancy. Thus abdominal crunches and situps are necessarily limited during pregnancy. Second, pushing during the second stage of labor is very fatiguing and it is easy to guess that women in good physical condition may have an advantage. While no scientific study has been made of this issue, this is where a small kernel of truth may lie in terms of the benefits of exercise. However, from my own observations of women in labor, motivation and self-discipline seem vastly more important than physical conditioning during the few hours of pushing. Perhaps the needed motivation and self-discipline comes in part through knowledge, which has made me a fan of childbirth classes. I personally do not feel that I can predict who will thrive during the second stage of labor no matter how well I know the patient.

Finally, there is much discussion about preparing the vaginal opening through stretching, massages with oil, and Kegel exercises. None of these activities have been scientifically studied so that their benefit remains unknown. (This is different than saying that they are known to be of no benefit; they may be helpful or even harmful—we simply do not know.) As a practical matter, it seems difficult to imagine that much can be done to assure comfort when the object emerging through the vaginal opening will be a bony structure (the baby's head) that is 4 inches in diameter with a 12.5-inch circumference.

In summary, pregnant women should maintain their exercise program to improve longevity and the quality of life. Pregnancy should not prevent someone from starting an exercise program with these goals in mind. However, it makes little sense to start exercising simply on the theory that labor will be easier as a result.

Myth #52:
Back labor is particularly uncomfortable.

This myth holds that labor primarily felt against one's back (as opposed to the front) is uniquely painful. While the notion is popular among the lay population and promulgated by some childbirth-class instructors, the idea has never been scientifically evaluated. As a result, I am forced to rely on my own observations of thousands of labors. It is my opinion that the degree of pain experienced in labor is so highly variable from woman to woman and pregnancy to pregnancy that it is difficult to generalize. Depending on the circumstances, labor can be extremely painful whether much of the sensation is experienced in the back or in the front. It should be noted that the statements here are speculative—no doubt some doctors would disagree with me. Yet until scientific study demonstrates otherwise, the concept that back labor is uniquely painful should be regarded with skepticism. The bogeyman of painful "back labor" serves to frighten expectant mothers unnecessarily—frightening them about something which has not been confirmed by any scientific observation.

Myth #53:
"Posterior" babies cause back labor.

Again this is a source of anxiety for expectant mothers in which the medical literature has little to say. The reference to "posterior" means that the fetal back is closer to the maternal back than the maternal abdominal wall. There is no evidence to support the idea that babies positioned this way will cause laboring mothers to experience more pain in the back than in the front.

MYTH #54:
Walking tends to help the progress of labor.

Hard as I have tried, I could find virtually no information on this issue in any obstetrical textbook. In a computer search of the literature, I could also find very little on the subject. In the meager information available, some investigators suggest that ambulation may help speed labor but others could find no such benefit. As a result, there is much room for doubt. At the present, the idea that walking (or gravity for that matter) influences the course of labor must be regarded as speculative. Of particular concern to me as an obstetrician is having a patient decline a medically appropriate recommendation for labor induction or augmentation on the theory that if she simply walks around longer, the speed of labor will be enhanced. Though ferociously promulgated by some, walking has simply not been clearly established as an efficacious way to hasten labor. Parenthetically, this is not to say that walking has no value. It does seem to be a good way to pass time in early labor and in this way some mothers certainly find it helpful.

MYTH #55:
Healing from a tear is less painful than
healing from an episiotomy (or vice versa).

Episiotomies have attracted much controversy in recent years. Do they help? Are they necessary? The issue that I wish to address is that of postpartum pain. It is my belief that the degree of pain experienced during recovery is completely unpredictable and is not influenced by whether a patient tears or has a so-called "surgical" incision. While it seems desirable to keep the tear or episiotomy to a minimum, I have found that some patients with small episiotomies have more pain than others who have torn all the way into their rectum.

In keeping with this personal observation, at least one study in the medical literature has confirmed my bias. In a study of 93 first-time mothers who experienced vaginal birth in Australia, the authors could find no difference in postpartum pain between those who had an episiotomy and those who did not. Of note is the fact that among the 35 women who did not receive an episiotomy, 24 required sutures anyway and 7 experienced tears that did not require stitches.

Delivery

MYTH #56:
Common hospital practice includes shaving pubic hairs and giving enemas in early labor.

I do not know when these practices stopped being commonplace, but it has been at least 15 years. For some reason, many classroom instructors feel compelled to make this a big issue. Yet in most institutions, pubic hairs are *never* shaved in ordinary circumstances and more patients (not many) request enemas than are offered them. Parenthetically, an enema in early labor may not be a bad idea for some women since any stool in the rectum will be pushed out during the birth process.

MYTH #57:
Vacuum and forceps deliveries are dangerous and should always be avoided.

In debunking this myth, it should be noted that obstetric practice has changed significantly over the past three decades. Rather than perform a difficult (and potentially dangerous) forceps delivery, obstetricians in current practice perform Cesarean sections. This may be one small reason why the Cesarean section rate has risen in recent times, though I cannot imagine anyone arguing against this specific change in practice. With the more complicated, instrument-aided vaginal delivery a thing of the past, forceps and vacuum use are very safe.

In general, the most common reason for offering assistance to the mother while pushing is a long second stage, in which maternal energy is fading fast and vaginal delivery seems to be a sure bet, given enough time. As a rule, this precludes assisting the birth of a fetus high in the pelvis or one who needs substantial rotation to "corkscrew" through the birth canal. The trend of deferring intervention until the fetus is lower in the birth canal has served to improve the safety of forceps and vacuum to the point that no specific increased risk of fetal injury has been consistently identified in outcome studies of these so-called operative deliveries. For instance, in one study of 32,000 17-year-olds, the average I.Q. of those delivered by forceps or vacuum was not different than those delivered vaginally without assistance or those delivered by cesarean.

Cesarean Delivery

Myth #58:
Fetal distress is the most common reason for Cesarean birth.

To clarify matters at the outset, there is no definition of fetal distress or a consensus on what the term means in the medical community. On the other hand, fetal intolerance to labor is generally taken to mean that if nothing changes, the fetus will suffer injury from oxygen deprivation if labor continues for a substantial length of time. If this concept seems somewhat vague, it is, and this is because we do not fully understand the relationship between neurologic injury and oxygen deprivation during labor. (Please also see the discussions regarding mental retardation and cerebral palsy on pages 94 and 95, respectively.)

As of the mid-1980s, the most common reason for Cesarean section was simply a history of Cesarean delivery with the previous pregnancy. This statistic may be changing as more and more doctors and patients are attempting a trial of labor in pregnancies following a Cesarean birth. The next most common reason (and probably by now, the largest single reason) to perform a Cesarean section, is failure to progress during labor. Fetal intolerance to labor is only the third most common reason for a Cesarean. The rates for the mid-1980s were as follows: for every 100 deliveries, there were 25 Cesarean sections, nine of which were due to repeat Cesarean, eight due to failure to progress, and two due to fetal intolerance. Phrased differently, while a woman without a prior Cesarean has roughly a one in six chance of Cesarean birth, the likelihood that she will need a Cesarean because the fetus experiences difficulty during labor is only one in 50.

MYTH #59:
A woman who has a history of genital herpes will require Cesarean delivery.

Genital herpes is the bane of the gynecologist's existence. It often causes patients more emotional distress than other sexually transmitted disease. This is quite strange to the medical practitioner who well knows that other sexually transmitted diseases, such as gonorrhea, chlamydia, and cervical warts potentially have much more adverse consequences. In fact, herpes has truly taken on the mythical qualities of a "dread disease." Upon closer examination, it is quite clear that patients who acquire herpes actually suffer very little injury. The virus does not cause infertility nor does it cause cancer, as once thought. It has no affect on health whatsoever other than the occasional appearance of painful blisters on the perineum. Repeat episodes are typically much less uncomfortable than the first.

In keeping with the legend of Herpes, many people have the mistaken notion that they will need Cesarean delivery. It is true that a herpes infection in the newborn is disastrous: at least half of the newborns die and approximately half of the survivors suffer permanent neurologic injury. However, at the present, the medical literature recommends Cesarean delivery only for women with visible genital sores at the time of labor or ruptured membranes. It has been estimated that only two to five percent of the population with a history of genital herpes will have an outbreak close to the time of labor. In practice, most women with genital herpes are able to deliver vaginally.

In most of the discussions regarding herpes in the medical literature, two generally accepted facts seem to be underemphasized.

First, the incidence of serious newborn herpes infections in the United States is approximately one in 10,000 (or equal to the maternal death rate and roughly half the risk of anyone dying in a car crash during one year of driving). Also, the majority of babies with herpes infections are actually born to mothers with no history of the disease and no sores at the time of delivery. Fortunately, neonatal herpes is quite rare whether or not the mother has a history of genital herpes and no matter what route of delivery is chosen.

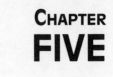

The Baby
Before, During,
and After Birth

Gender Prediction

MYTH #60:
The fetal heart rate provides a clue about gender.

No matter how many times I deny it, patients and their husbands remain convinced that somehow I know the gender of the baby. The focus of most of these fantasies is, of course, the fetal heart rate. Interestingly enough, I myself cannot keep the myth straight. I do not know if a "fast" heartbeat means a girl or boy. In fact, I do not know the definition of a "fast" heartbeat in this context. Nonetheless, the best way to demolish this myth is to momentarily accept its basic premise as true. What if fetal boys and girls did have different average heart rates as a group? Could checking the heart rate in the office or at home predict gender better than guessing?

The first bit of bad news for believers is that it has been proven that doctors cannot accurately determine the heart rate from simply listening to it. In a study in which 15 obstetricians were asked to determine heart rate from a variety of prerecorded heartbeats, there was a wide range of variation. By the time the heart rate reached 180 beats per minute, the estimates were as much as 60 beats per minute different from each other. Therefore it is clear that without an actual computerized count (rarely done in the office), the fetal heart rate cannot be accurately determined. As a result, defining the rate as fast or slow is inaccurate, and this observation is meaningless in predicting gender even if boys and girls had different heart rates. Parenthetically, the fetal heartbeat is checked in the office primarily for presence or absence—not rate.

Return now to the initial premise that there is a difference in the average heart rate between fetal boys and girls. For the sake of argument, let us imagine a study in which the heart rate of 10,000 fetal boys and 10,000 fetal girls were studied for six hours at 32 weeks. (In such a study, gender would be assigned retrospectively at the time of birth.) Further, let us say that the study found an average heart rate for boys of 142 and for girls of 138. On this basis could one predict the gender for Mrs. Jones's baby? In a word, no. Some boys would have average heart rates of 130 while some girls would have average heart rates of 150. Even if the averages were different, there would be so much overlap between the two groups that gender prediction in the case of a specific baby would be little better than flipping a coin.

Additional factors make gender prediction even more hopeless. Fetal heartbeats are well known to change from one minute to the next. In fact, this variability is so well characterized that it is classified as "short-term" and "long-term." Even if one could accurately determine the count from one minute of listening, the value would change depending on when one took the rate. Also, the average fetal heart rate is known to slowly decline over the course of the third trimester. The same baby would be expected to have a different heart rate at 36 weeks from that taken at 28 weeks.

Of course, there is no study to my knowledge that has even tried to assess the gender difference in fetal heart rates. In fact, in an entire book on fetal monitoring, I could find no reference to gender in the index nor was there a single reference to gender in the entire text! So for those who state that there is a difference in heart rates by gender, my reply is that this is not known to be true. (To be precise, it is also not known to be false since my fantasy study above has never been performed.) Yet even if this gender difference were proven to be true, it would not matter, since: 1) doctors cannot determine the rate accurately from just listening in the office, 2) if such a difference did exist, there would be so much overlap in the rates between the genders that prediction would still not be accurate, 3) the heart rate of a single fetus changes greatly from moment to moment, and 4) the average heart rate for babies is known to drop over time.

MYTH #61:
The way a mother carries gives a clue to gender.

As with the heart-rate myth, I am not clear on the specifics—that is, does a mother who carries "high" have a greater chance for a boy or a girl? The answer to this question does not matter because a woman's external appearance provides no clue as to the gender contained within.

A pregnant woman's physical appearance (and the way she appears to be carrying) is dependent on five obvious characteristics. These are: 1) height, 2) starting weight, 3) weight gain, 4) skeletal structure, and 5) length of the gestation. As should be obvious, none of these factors are associated with fetal gender.

MYTH #62:
Heartburn means it is a boy (or a girl).

Though I have heard this statement dozens of times, here too, I do not remember which gender is supposedly predicted. Suffice it to say, that as with the myths above, this is simply not true. Heart-burn is a common symptom of pregnancy and is thought to occur both because emptying of the stomach is known to slow in pregnant women, and because in the third trimester, the uterus provides significant upward pressure on the stomach. The over-the-counter antiacids are safe to use and can be particularly helpful at bedtime when this condition is typically worse.

MYTH #63:

The Chinese birthing chart can predict gender more accurately than guessing.

A Chicago radio station has recently distributed a "Chinese birthing chart." For one dollar (that is contributed to charity), the station will send out this guide to gender prediction. I had already seen this chart many times over the years when patients brought them in.

"This chart has been taken from a Royal Tomb near Peking, China. A Chinese scientist discovered the chart, which had been buried in the tomb for 700 years. The original copy is kept in the Institute of Science of Peking." The accuracy of the chart is *claimed* to have been proven by thousands of people and is believed to be 99 percent accurate. Parenthetically, this claim exceeds the most optimistic assessments of ultrasound accuracy in determining gender.

The chart then instructs the reader. "Find the sex of your unborn child by checking the mother's age when she gives birth (vertical rows) and the month of conception (horizontal rows)."

When I see nonsense like this, I wonder if I should have chosen a different career. To take but one example, if the mother will be age 31 at birth, the gender prediction based on the month of conception (January through December) is as follows: M/F/F/F/F/F/F/F/F/F/F/M. Fortunately, the pranksters that made this chart up were mathematically illiterate and their work can be debunked with a simple glance. With the simplifying assumption that the monthly birth rate is approximately the same throughout the year, it can be seen that mothers delivering at age 31 will give birth to males only if they conceived in January or December. This chart therefore predicts that as a group, women who are 31 when they deliver will give birth to girls 10 out of 12 times or 83.3 percent of the time. The idea that women 31 years old will give birth to girls 83.3 percent of the time is clearly nonsense, as is the Chinese Birth Chart.

In a sense, the "Chinese Birth Chart" is a disappointing hoax. Had the chart designers been slightly more sophisticated, they could have made a chart that would predict 50 percent males and females for each maternal birth age. That would have been a little more difficult to debunk.

MYTH #64:
Having sex before ovulation increases the chance of a boy.

This myth has proven to be quite a vexation for me since it has led to some unexpected findings. First, there may be more than a kernel of truth in it (but how can I count it as a myth if it is not a myth?). Second, it also seems that deliberately trying to conceive in advance of or after ovulation may be associated with an increased risk of birth defects. Thus the subject is much more complicated than it would first appear.

All the information on the relationship between coitus and time of ovulation comes not from studies of people trying to affect gender but rather studies of contraceptive failures in the course of practicing natural family planning or periodic abstinence. The whole basis for efficacy of this method is avoiding intercourse when a women is fertile. Therefore, there is considerable scientific interest in evaluating the pregnancy outcomes of pregnancies that occur in spite of this method.

There is preliminary evidence that conceptions that take place from coitus two days or so in advance of ovulation are more likely to produce males than from intercourse which has taken place very close to ovulation. At the same time, there is also theoretical speculation along with a smattering of data that conceptions that occur from coitus remote from ovulation may be associated with an increased risk of miscarriage and birth defects. For the present, two conclusions seem warranted. There may be truth in the idea that having intercourse in advance of ovulation may slightly increase the odds of having a boy. It may also be true that deliberately changing behavior to accomplish this may also be increasing the risk of miscarriage or birth defects. While the final verdict is not yet in, it seems that "It's not nice to fool mother nature."

Fetal Health

Myth #65:
It is a good idea to interview pediatricians
to decide on which one to use.

The views presented here are strictly opinion and not medical fact. However, they can serve as a useful balance for those books and health professionals who advocate interviewing pediatricians to help decide whom to use.

As with so many things in life, such as career selection, choice of college, and even picking a spouse, decisions have to be made on the basis of incomplete information. Many people are made exceedingly uncomfortable by this fact. Unfortunately, many more are not even aware of this truth. Even a relatively small decision, such as doctor selection, has to be made in the absence of a complete set of facts. In other words, the choice is somewhat arbitrary and subject to chance.

Four obvious and objective characteristics of a pediatrician help narrow the selection process. He or she should be board certified, have admitting privileges at the hospital at which you plan to deliver, and have an office fairly convenient to your home. An increasingly important issue, of course, is whether or not the doctor is in your insurance plan. Does interviewing the doctor beforehand increase the probability that you will be happy with your pediatric care? I suggest not.

Pediatricians, as well as all of their colleagues in other specialties, have technical training, focusing on science and patient care. They are not businessmen, sales people, or public speakers. The interview process, in which a patient queries the pediatrician with the sole purpose of deciding whether or not to use that doctor subsequently, is a highly atypical and artificial situation for the physician. Like it or not, the doctor is under some compulsion to "sell" himself. This is a very uncomfortable setting for many. As such, it is predictable that there is no meaningful relationship between the doctor's interview performance and his or her behavior in the more natural doctor/patient setting.

This in fact has been my experience with my patients who interview pediatricians. Some pleasant, mild-mannered doctors appear surly while other doctors who are not especially eager-to-please

are positively charming during the interview. I advise my patients
to use the four criteria described above and see how things go.
Most doctors in private practice could not stay in practice if they
did not provide appropriate care and please the vast majority of
their patients.

MYTH #66:
Having the umbilical cord wound around the baby's neck is a major cause of newborn death and injury.

This myth is the source of considerable concern among expectant parents. Some even go so far as to suggest that we do an ultrasound at term just to be sure this is not the case. (As it turns out,
ultrasound is not very reliable in detecting this condition.) Birth
with the umbilical cord around the neck is actually a commonplace
event—occurring in 25% of all live births. This situation is simply
not dangerous or known to cause injury.

While at first glance this statement makes no sense, it is important to remember that the fetus actually breathes through
the umbilical cord, so the fetus cannot choke if its neck is
squeezed. There is blood flow to the neck but it is relatively limited in that it is simply supplying the brain. As I often tell my
patients, having the cord around the neck is like wrapping a garden
hose around a fire hydrant. Trying to stop the flow through the
hose by wrapping it tightly around the hydrant is very difficult
indeed. In fact, I can recall delivering a healthy baby with the
umbilical cord wrapped around its neck *four* times. It was so tight
that I couldn't even put clamps across it before I cut it. In another
case, I delivered a baby with both cord around the neck and a true
knot in the umbilical cord. This newborn was also perfectly

healthy. As can be seen, even in these extreme circumstances, it is very hard to choke the fetus, either at the neck or by compressing the umbilical cord.

MYTH #67:
The baby's movements tend to slow down right before labor.

This statement is simply wrong. I do not know where it originated, but it is a widely held belief. It is very disturbing because, in at least a few cases, fetuses who are quite sick actually stop or slow their movements for a few days before death. For this reason, obstetricians often ask patients to call if they notice a substantial decrease in fetal movement from one day to the next.

As this issue causes much confusion, some clarification is in order. First, decreased fetal movement as a symptom of fetal illness is admittedly rare. Expectant mothers often call us with complaints of decreased movement and further evaluation almost always establishes that the fetus is in good health. Nonetheless, a large change in the pattern of movement (i.e., decrease) over a 12- to-24-hour period of time is worth a call to the obstetrician.

A common observation of patients that does not seem to appear in obstetric texts is that the quality of fetal movement does indeed seem to change for many over time. It may be less vigorous or kicks may be replaced by rolls. In terms of monitoring movements, pregnant woman should not be comparing this month to last month but rather today with yesterday and the day before. A large decrease in the number of movements as opposed to their strength or nature is worth a call to the doctor.

Finally, coming back to the myth itself, while it is true that healthy fetuses may change their movement pattern in a short period of time, there is simply no truth to the idea that any change in fetal behavior is related to the onset of labor.

Myth #68:
The Apgar score is an important predictor of the baby's health.

In responding to this statement, I never asked for or knew the Apgar scores of any of my three children. The Apgar score is an on-the-spot assessment of the newborn's breathing efforts, heart beat, cry, tone, and color. As such, it is meant to provide a formal guide to the medical staff about caring for the newborn in the first five minutes of life. It simply does not predict fetal health afterward and is not a clue to intelligence or anything else. As a general rule, if the baby is crying and moving within the first few minutes of birth, it is fine. This is what I call the eyeball, across-the-room Apgar score, and as the father or the obstetrician, it is the one I use most often. Parenthetically, as most babies are bluish or purple in the first five minutes of life, the British do not even include newborn color in their assessment system.

Myth #69:
Streptococcus is a particularly dangerous bacteria and is a common cause of newborn injury and death.

This myth got started because, on rare occasions, Group B Streptococcus (GBS) can cause injury or death to newborns. Because of media attention, the disease has inspired more anxiety that the facts and statistics would seem to warrant.

GBS is so commonly present that it can be regarded as a normal inhabitant of the vagina. Depending on the study, figures show that 15 to 40 percent of pregnant women are colonized—that is, they carry the bacteria in their body without any evidence of disease. Of those colonized, the numbers of bacteria seem to vary over time insofar as serial cultures will be intermittently negative, even in the absence of treatment.

Among those infants that do become ill, there is an early-onset and late-onset syndrome. Early-onset illness occurs within seven days of birth, though more than half of these babies demonstrate illness within six hours of birth. Symptoms generally derive from sepsis (so-called blood poisoning), pneumonia, or meningitis. Unfortunately, the illness can be so sudden and severe that up to 15 percent of newborns with early-onset disease die. Late-onset disease typically appears as meningitis more than a week after birth. In both types of GBS infection, it is believed that the infant acquires the bacteria directly from the mother during birth in half of the cases.

Clearly, GBS can cause serious problems for newborns. But just how common is it? The overall rate for early-onset disease is only one to three per 1,000 births. (In comparison, the overall risk for birth defects is on the order of 20 to 30 per 1,000 births.) Late-onset disease is somewhat less common. Among the 40 percent of the population that is colonized, the rate is only ten per 1,000. In other words, even if a mother is known to have GBS in the vagina, her risk for newborn infection is only 1 percent.

Can anything be done to reduce the chance of newborn infection? While several strategies have been proposed to help prevent newborn illness, the one that seems to make the most sense is simply administering antibiotics (typically penicillin) during labor to mothers with known risk factors such as fever during labor or prolonged rupture of membranes. As the antibiotic does indeed cross the placenta to reach the baby, the rate of newborn infection has been shown to drop with the treatment of laboring women with known risk factors. There is controversy about the benefits of culturing women before labor because it does not seem likely to be beneficial since, as a practical matter, newborn GBS infection is an unlikely complication of childbirth. The current practice of antibiotic treatment for mothers at particular risk can make this illness even more uncommon.

Birth Defects

MYTH #70:
A normal ultrasound excludes birth defects.

Even with great improvements in ultrasound technology over the past decade, a normal ultrasound does not guarantee a normal baby. Many genetic problems that can lead to severe or even fatal problems for the newborn such as Tay-Sachs disease or sickle-cell anemia do not cause anatomical abnormalities. Many anatomical problems may not be very evident in the middle trimester when ultrasounds are done. Finally, they can simply be hard to detect even when present. For example, reports published from university centers suggest that 20 to 50 percent of fetuses with serious heart defects will be missed by ultrasound. It's sad to say, but what has been true since humans first evolved remains true today: no one can be guaranteed a normal, healthy baby, no matter what tests are done.

MYTH #71:
A leading cause of mental retardation is lack of oxygen during labor.

This myth has its roots in the medical community. In fact, this was such a firmly held belief that continuous electronic fetal monitoring was widely introduced before (and in the absence of) any evidence that it could reduce the rate of neonatal neurologic injury. Severe mental retardation occurs at the rate of about 3.5 per 1,000 population while mild mental retardation is predictably more common at the rate of 23 to 31 per 1,000. It is now estimated that only 5 to 10 percent of individuals with mental retardation suffered a critical injury during the childbirth process. Even more compelling, in longterm studies of babies thought to have had oxygen deprivation at birth, the vast majority (greater than 90 percent) of them were subsequently found to be of normal intelligence.

MYTH #72:
A leading cause of cerebral palsy is lack of oxygen during labor.

Cerebral palsy is defined as a "chronic neuromuscular disability characterized by aberrant control of movement or posture, appearing early in life and not the result of recognized progressive disease." Cerebral palsy may be complicated by a seizure disorder or mental retardation. Premature birth is the leading suspected factor in these cases, although the causes of the disease remain poorly understood. In one study of 189 children with cerebral palsy, suspected lack of oxygen during delivery was the suspected cause in only 21 (roughly 10 percent). Conversely, other studies have found that 90 percent of people with cerebral palsy did not have oxygen deprivation during the birth process. It has also been suggested that babies with preexisting neurological injury may display abnormal heart-rate patterns during labor, creating the false impression that oxygen deprivation may have caused the brain damage when in fact it was already present before labor. Finally, the rate of cerebral palsy occurrence—one to two cases per 1,000—has not changed in the past 20 years in the United States despite a rising Cesarean section rate or widespread use of continuous electronic fetal monitoring.

MYTH #73:
Medical X rays pose a significant threat to the fetus and should always be avoided.

There are two separate potential dangers from ionizing radiation (the type of energy used in medical X rays): an increased rate of birth defects and cancer. Data has been obtained from animal studies, atomic bomb survivors, and pregnant women who received medical X rays. The fetus is most susceptible to neurologic damage from radiation during the 8 to 15 weeks after the first day of the last menstrual period. Nonetheless, the data is conclusive in that the amount of radiation involved in a single diagnostic study does not increase the risk of birth defects at any time in the pregnancy. An important exception to the safety of medical X rays during pregnancy is the use of multiple studies, particularly during the most susceptible period at the end of the first trimester and start of the second trimester. X ray effects are thought to be cumulative.

One particular concern that frequently arises is that of dental X rays. Since the X ray beam is focused at the skull, the amount of radiation to the fetus is extremely small indeed. As explained above, even X ray studies of the maternal abdomen during pregnancy are thought to be perfectly safe as long as only one diagnostic test is done (this typically involves a series of X rays taken during one occasion).

The second issue, an increased risk of cancer after birth, is somewhat less well understood. At the present, it is believed that there may be an increased risk of childhood leukemia at radiation doses encountered in the most intensive type of diagnostic studies such as abdominal CAT scans. In this context, it has been estimated that the rate of childhood leukemia might increase by an additional one per 6,000 people. It should be pointed out that the dose of radiation in most medical X rays is much less. For instance, the dose of radiation used in a traditional abdominal study is 5 to 30 times less. For a mammogram or chest X ray, the amount of radiation is a tiny fraction of that used in a CAT scan (more than 100 times less). With this in mind, there are many settings in which the benefits of medical X rays far outweigh any conceivable disadvantage. These include virtually all reasons: dental X rays, abdominal X rays for maternal trauma, and even X rays to determine the presentation or position of the fetus (i.e., in the case of breech babies or twins).

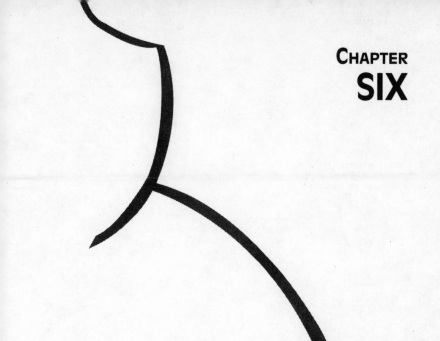

*A*fter
the Birth

Recovery

MYTH #74:

**Childbirth scars are a common cause of
painful intercourse long after the birth.**

In the only study that I could find on the subject involving the follow-up of 93 patients, only 20 percent were still having discomfort during intercourse six months after the delivery. Almost all of these patients were free of pain by 12 months postpartum. These statistics seem to confirm my experience in private practice—childbirth events are simply not a common cause of longstanding painful intercourse.

MYTH #75:

**Women cannot get pregnant again
before their first postpartum period.**

My partners and I warn every single patient who delivers that they can become pregnant again immediately. The typical reply is, "Oh, you don't have to worry about that, Dr. Benson." Taken literally, the reply is peculiar since it would never occur to me to worry about whether or not a specific patient gets pregnant. In this area, we like to leave the worrying to the patients. Unfortunately, some do not take our counselling to heart. Every year we deliver a few babies before their sibling turns one. Since this is almost always very distressing to the couples, it is wise to use condoms or some other contraceptive device with every episode of postpartum intercourse if it is not the couple's objective to have another child immediately. Women can and do ovulate within a few weeks of delivery on occasion. This can occur before a woman has the first period after delivery.

MYTH #76:
Postpartum "blues" are widely experienced after delivery and are often severe and long lasting.

The symptoms of postpartum blues include depressed mood, crying spells, irritability, anxiety, mood swings, confusion, and sleep and appetite disturbance. While the frequency of this problem varies considerably according to the medical literature, these symptoms are reasonably common and probably occur in about one-fourth of the population. If crying alone is measured, up to 85 percent of the population can be said to have postpartum blues. This sort of mild depression has been attributed to the emotional letdown after delivery, the pain of postpartum recovery, sleep deprivation, anxieties over caring for the newborn, and worries over her relationship with her mate. Nonetheless, the majority of mothers do not have a full-blown episode of the blues. Fortunately, this sort of mild depression lasts only a few days, although it can persist for up to ten days.

The self-limited and mild nature of the "blues" usually makes medical attention unnecessary. It is important to emphasize that this problem should only be mild and short-lived. Thoughts about suicide and persistence of symptoms beyond a week or ten days are strongly suggestive of depression, and if this occurs a physician should be consulted.

MYTH #77:

Women with postpartum depression will make bad mothers because they really do not want their babies.

This is a particularly sad myth because it blames the victim for an illness over which she has no control. In recent years it has become quite clear that depression is largely a chemically mediated change in the brain. People are often genetically predisposed to such changes but overwhelming environmental circumstances can bring about depression in a person who may not have an underlying predisposition. It has been estimated that approximately 10 percent of the population by six weeks postpartum suffers from depression. Of note is the fact that postpartum depression is not different in symptoms and treatment from depression occurring at other times in a woman's life. In fact, most medical studies suggest that the rate of depression in the postpartum period is actually the same as depression at other periods of life.

With regard to the patient's fitness for motherhood, as long as the depression is treated and she responds, there is simply no reason to believe that she will have particular difficulties as a parent. Although many parents may be ambivalent about their new responsibilities, depression per se should not be taken as a rejection of either the baby or the mother's new role. Instead, it should be emphasized that a certain percentage of the population is depressed from time to time and the postpartum period does not make women immune to this malady.

Nursing

MYTH #78:

Mothers who nurse cannot get pregnant.

As with some of myths in this book, there is a small element of truth in this statement. The infertility conferred by nursing is simply not reliable enough for individuals determined to avoid pregnancy. There are some general truths regarding nursing and fertility:

1. Nursing delays the return of ovulation.

2. The longer a woman nurses, the more likely ovulation and menstruation will return while she is nursing.

3. The longer she nurses, the more likely it is that ovulation will precede the first period.

From the above, it should be clear that nursing and absence of menses does not guarantee infertility. Another consideration is the fact that the menstrual cycle is commonly irregular during nursing and the diagnosis of pregnancy may therefore be delayed.

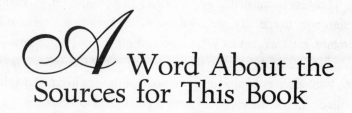 Word About the Sources for This Book

There are four sources that I used regularly, but because some of the myths were relatively obscure, I turned to computerized searches using Medline. This is a database in which the titles and abstracts of papers appearing in thousands of medical journals are entered into a massive computerized log. By specifying the topic of interest, the computer can generate a list of articles on the subject. Of course, the articles produced by the search are highly dependent on the particular terminology used. Thus, a search done on the same subject by two different people can yield different article lists. Also, on many subjects, conflicting reports can be found. In citing the medical literature from computer searches, I tried to present a consensus view as I saw it. Unfortunately, on many of these subjects, the last word has not been written. It is possible, if not unlikely, that the myth of today will be fact tomorrow (or even the reverse).

With regard to my four principal sources, it is worth noting that these references are updated very regularly. Also, in citing them, I tried not to take facts out of context and chose to use only those that I felt represented a widespread medical consensus. A few words about each source is in order.

1. Cunningham, G. F., MacDonald, P. C., Gant, N. F., Leveno, K. J., Gilstrap, III, L. C. *Williams Obstetrics, 19th edition.* Norwalk, Connecticut: Appleton and Lange, 1993.

This text is unusually well written and documented. It contains references to literally several thousand articles in the medical literature. First written by Whitridge J. Williams in 1902, a new edition has been published on the average of every five years. Though the book does not cover every topic in obstetrics in equal depth or with equal accuracy, it does have much useful information.

It is designated in the reference section as *Williams*.

2. American College of Obstetricians and Gynecologists (ACOG) Technical Bulletins.

Published monthly by ACOG, these bulletins are meant to provide guidance on specific subjects. Not intended to be applicable in all cases, they nonetheless have practical utility. Typically as a new bulletin on a particular subject is published, an old one is designated as outdated and meant to be discarded. In this way, ACOG keeps the number of current bulletins relatively fixed and assures a continuous updating progress as new knowledge is acquired.

3. Sciarra, J. J., ed. *Gynecology and Obstetrics*. Philadelphia: J.B. Lippincott Company, 1994.

This is a unique creation—a six-volume loose-leaf text. The company publishes new chapters every year along with instructions to discard chapters that have become outdated. With approximately 550 chapters and over 500 authors, it contains several thousand references as does *Williams*. Parenthetically, Dr. Sciarra was Chairman of the Department of Obstetrics and Gynecology while I was a resident at Northwestern. He continues in that position today.

It is designated in reference section as *Sciarra*.

4. Creasy, R. K., Resnik, R. *Maternal-Fetal Medicine: Principles and Practice, 3rd edition*. Philadelphia: W.B. Saunders Company, 1994.

With over 70 contributors, this textbook also contains thousands of references. Dr. Creasy is department chairman at the University of Texas in Houston and Dr. Resnik is department chairman at the University of California, San Diego.

It is designated in the reference section as *Creasy and Resnik*.

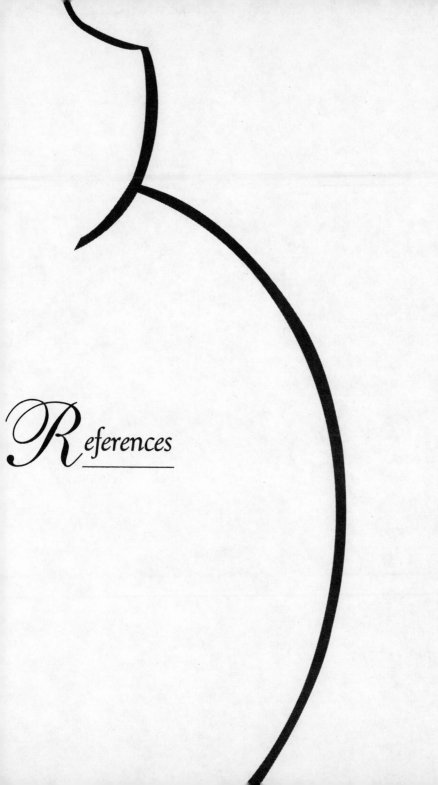

References

CHAPTER ONE:

Myths of Conception and The First Trimester

High Risk

MYTH #1: A pregnant woman age 35 or over is at "high risk."

1. Global risk assessment in the 1960s.
   Sciarra. Dombrowski, M.P. and Sokol R.J. "Risk Assessment and the Perinatal Database." Vol. 3, Ch. 2.
   Sciarra. Depp, R. "Care of the High Risk Mother." Vol. 3, Ch. 1.
2. Maternal death rate, illness rates, fetal outcomes as a function of age.
   Williams. "Pregnancy at the Extremes of Reproductive Life." Ch. 30, pp. 653–9.
3. Genetic statements.
   A. Overall rate of birth defects.
      Sciarra. Pergament, E. "Cytogenetics." Vol. 5, Ch. 73, p. 23. (20% of all birth defects—0.65%, 3% overall rate)
   B. Age and risk of chromosome errors.
      Simpson J. L., Golbus, M.S., Martin, A.O., Sarto, G.E.

Genetics in Obstetrics and Gynecology. New York: Grune and Stratton, 1982, p. 58. (age and risk of chromosome errors)

C. Amniocentesis risk.
Simpson, J.L., Golbus, M.S., Martin A.O., Sarto, G.E. *Genetics in Obstetrics and Gynecology.* New York: Grune and Stratton, 1982, p. 110. (amniocentesis risk)

Miscarriage

MYTH #5: Cramping in early pregnancy is a warning signal for miscarriage.

1. No reference in texts to cramping in early pregnancy.
   Creasy and Resnik. Glass, R.H. and Golbus, M.S. "Recurrent Abortion." Ch. 29, p. 446.
   Sciarra. McNeeley, J.R., S.J. "Early Abortion." Vol. 2, ch. 23, p. 2.
   Williams. "Abortion." Ch. 31, p. 676.

MYTH #6: Cramping in early pregnancy is an indication that an ectopic pregnancy has occurred.

1. Incidence of ectopic pregnancy is one in 100.
   Williams. "Ectopic pregnancy." Ch. 32, p. 693.

MYTH #7: Vigorous exercise increases the risk of miscarriage.

1. Maternal heating during exercise not dangerous.
   Howard, H. and Mitchell, B. "Atmospheric Variations, Noise, and Vibration." Ch. 16, p. 220. In: Paul, M., ed. *Occupational and Environmental Reproductive Hazards: A Guide For Clinicians.* Baltimore: Williams and Wilkins, 1993.

MYTH #8: Falling can cause miscarriages.

1. Falling dismissed as cause of miscarriages.
   Williams. "Abortion." Ch. 31, p. 672.

MYTH #9: A woman who miscarries always (or never) needs a D and C.

1. Classification of miscarriages.
   Sciarra. McNeeley, Jr., G. "Early Abortion." Vol. 2, ch. 23, p. 4.

MYTH #10: Hormone imbalances are a common cause of miscarriages.

1. Incidence and diagnosis of progesterone deficiency.
   Williams. "Abortion." Ch. 31, pp. 668–9.

MYTH #11: A woman who miscarries is actually fortunate because the baby would have been abnormal.

1. Chromosome errors are common cause of miscarriage.
   Williams. "Abortion." Ch. 31, p. 667.

Early Symptoms

MYTH #13: Women with severe morning sickness are trying to "vomit out the pregnancy."

1. Stress and nausea of pregnancy.
   Williams. "Gastrointestinal Disorders." Ch. 51, p. 1146.
   Sciarra. Anderson, G.D. "Nutrition in Pregnancy." Vol. 2, ch. 7, pp. 11–12.

CHAPTER TWO:

Nutrition and Medication

MYTH #14: Fruit juice is the drink of choice for a pregnant woman.

1. Calories of orange juice.
   Package labeling, Tropicana premium orange juice.
2. Calories in a pound of fat.
   Pemberton, C.M., Moxness, K.E., German, M.J., Nelson, J.K., Gastineau, C.F. *Mayo Clinic Diet Manual, 6th edition.* Toronto: B.C. Decker Inc., 1988, p. 6.
3. Calories in Coca-Cola and an orange.
   Pennington, J.A.T. *Bowes and Church's Food Values of Portions Commonly Used, 15th edition.* New York: Harper-Perennial, 1989, pp. 5, 99.

MYTH #15: Nutrasweet is not safe for pregnant women.

1. Facts on metabolism of Nutrasweet.
   London, R.S. "Saccharin and Aspartame: Are They Safe to Consume During Pregnancy?" *Journal of Reproductive Medicine.* 33:17–21. 1988.
   Council Report. "Aspartame: Review of Safety Issues." *Journal of the American Medical Association.* 254:400–2. 1985.
   Butchko, H.H. and Kotsonis, F.N. "Acceptable Daily Intake vs. Actual Intake: The Aspartame Example." *Journal of the American College of Nutrition.* 10:258–66. 1991.
   Kotsonis, F.N. and Butchko, H.H. "Aspartame: Review of Recent Research." *Comments Toxicology.* 3:253–78. 1989.

Filer, Jr., L.J. and Stegink, L.D. "Aspartame Metabolism in Normal Adults, Phenylketonuric Heterozygotes, and Diabetic Subjects." *Diabetes Care.* 12:67–74. 1989.

Stegink, L.D., Filer, Jr., L.J., Baker, G.L. "Plasma, Erythrocyte and Human Milk Levels of Free Amino Acids in Lactating Women Administered Aspartame, or Lactose." *Journal of Nutrition.* 1979. 109:2173–81.

Horwitz, D.L., McLane, M., Kobe, P. "Response to Single Dose of Aspartame or Saccharin by NIDDM Patients." *Diabetes Care.* 11:230–4. 1988.

2. Obesity linked to increased risk of gestational diabetes.
Naeye, R.L. "Maternal Body Weight and Pregnancy Outcome." *American Journal of Clinical Nutrition.* 52:273–9. 1990.

3. Abnormal weight gain linked to higher risk of Cesarean.
Ekblad, U. and Grenman, S. "Maternal Weight, Weight Gain during Pregnancy and Pregnancy Outcome." *International Journal of Gynaecology and Obstetrics.* 39:277–83. 1992.

Johnson, J.W., Longmate, J.A., Grentzen, R. "Excessive Maternal Weight and Pregnancy Outcome." *American Journal of Obstetrics and Gynecology.* 167:353–70. 1992.

MYTH #16: Prenatal vitamins are very important diet supplements.

1. Definition of vitamins.
Stedman's Medical Dictionary, 23rd edition. Baltimore: Williams & Wilkins, 1976, p. 1564.

2. Vitamin C of no benefit for colds.
Williams. "Prenatal Care." Ch. 9, p. 261.

3. Prenatal vitamins unnecessary.
Williams. "Prenatal Care." Ch. 9, p. 259.

Creasy and Resnik. Abrams, B. "Maternal Nutrition." Ch. 11, p. 166.
4. CDC recommendations.
   Creasy and Resnik. Abrams, B. "Maternal Nutrition." Ch. 11, p. 166.

MYTH #17: Pregnant women should not take medicine.

1. First week is protected.
   Simpson, J.L., Golbus, M.S., Martin, A.O., Sarto, G.E., *Genetics in Obstetrics and Gynecology.* New York: Grune and Stratton, 1982, p. 203.
2. Sulfa drugs and jaundice.
   Williams. "Drugs and Medications During Pregnancy." Ch. 42, p. 962.
3. 30 known teratogens.
   Williams. "Drugs and Medications During Pregnancy." Ch. 42, p. 960.
4. Asthma medication safe.
   Williams. "Drugs and Medications During Pregnancy." Ch. 42, p. 966.

MYTH #18: It is okay for a pregnant woman to have an occasional drink of alcohol.

1. All facts cited regarding alcohol consumption during pregnancy.
   Williams. "Drugs and Medications During Pregnancy." Ch. 42, p. 973–4.

CHAPTER THREE:
Middle and Late Pregnancy

Prenatal Screening

MYTH #19: Since the AFP test has a high false positive rate, it should be refused.

1. All factual information.
   "Alpha-Fetoprotein." *ACOG Technical Bulletin.* No. 154. April 1991.

MYTH #21: An abnormal screening test for diabetes strongly suggests that the patient has diabetes.

1. All statistics cited.
   Williams. "Endocrine Disorders." Ch. 53, p. 1205.
2. Controversy regarding screening.
   Creasy and Resnik. Moore, T.R. "Diabetes In Pregnancy." Ch. 54, p. 968.

Activity

MYTH #22: Pregnant women should use care not to sleep on their backs.

1. Review article.
   Kinsella, S.M. and Lohmann, G. "Review: Supine Hypotensive Syndrome." *Obstetrics and Gynecology.* 83:774–88. 1994.
2. Study of sleep positions in third trimester.
   Mills, G.H. and Chaffe, A.G. "Sleeping Positions Adopted by Pregnant Women of More Than 30 Weeks Gestation." *Anaesthesia.* 49:249–50. March 1994.

MYTH #23: Pregnant women should not exercise.

1. All data cited.

    "Exercise During Pregnancy and the Postpartum Period."
    ACOG Technical Bulletin. No. 189. February 1994.

MYTH #25: Lifting heavy objects can damage the baby.

1. General physical effort associated with preterm labor.

    Marbury, M.C. "Ergonomics." Ch. 15, pp. 201–17. In: Paul,
    M., ed. *Occupational and Environmental Reproductive Haz-
    ards: A Guide For Clinicians.* Baltimore: Williams and
    Wilkins, 1993.

Environmental Dangers

MYTH #27: Hot baths are dangerous for the fetus.

1. Pregnant women cannot tolerate rises in core temperature with-
    out discomfort.
2. Medical consensus is to not stay in sauna or hot tub for more
    than 15 minutes at a time.

    Hu, H. and Besser, M. "Atmospheric Variations, Noise, and
    Vibration." Ch. 16. pp. 218–20. In: Paul, M., ed., *Occupa-
    tional and Environmental Reproductive Hazards: A Guide
    For Clinicians.* Baltimore: Williams and Wilkins, 1993.

**MYTH #28: Do not let children play in the sandbox for fear of
toxoplasmosis.**

1. All factual information.

    "Perinatal Viral and Parasitic Infections." *ACOG Technical
    Bulletin.* No. 177. February 1993.

MYTH #29: Pregnant women should not perm their hair.

1. All factual information.

    Paul, M. "Common Household Exposures." Ch. 26, p. 367. IN: Paul, M., ed. *Occupational and Environmental Reproductive Hazards: A Guide For Clinicians.* Baltimore: Williams and Wilkins, 1993.

Symptoms

MYTH #30: Preeclampsia occurs in 20 percent of pregnancies.

1. Preeclampsia occurs in about 5 percent of the population.

    Williams. "Hypertensive disorders in pregnancy." Ch. 36, p. 767.

MYTH #31: A pregnant woman who has swelling probably has preeclampsia.

1. Swelling is not useful in diagnosing preeclampsia as it is too commonplace.

    Williams. "Hypertensive disorders in Pregnancy." Ch. 36, p. 764.

MYTH #33: Leg cramps are a symptom of blood clots.

1. Clots are rare.

    Williams. "Pulmonary Disorders." Ch. 49, p. 1112.

MYTH #34: Leg cramps are caused by a lack of calcium.

1. Double-blind study testing the role of calcium in leg cramps of pregnant women.

    Hammar, M., Berg, G., Soheim, F., Larsson, I. "Calcium and Magnesium Status in Pregnant Women. A Comparison Between Treatment with Calcium and Vitamin C in Pregnant

Women with Leg Cramps." *International Journal for Vitamin and Nutrition Research.* 57:179–83. 1987.

Preparing for and Predicting Labor

MYTH #35: It is possible to predict a woman's labor pattern from knowing her mother's labor pattern.

1. Success of vaginal birth after Cesarean for "failure to progress."

    Williams. "Cesarean Section and Cesarean Hysterectomy." Ch. 26, p. 596.

MYTH #36: Braxton Hicks contractions are different than labor contractions.

1. Who are Doctors Braxton and Hicks?
    Williams. "Maternal Adaptation to Pregnancy." Ch. 8, p. 210.
2. Labor definition.

    Friedman, E.A. *Labor: Clinical Evaluation and Management.* 2nd edition. New York: Appleton-Century-Crofts, 1978, p. 3.
3. Braxton Hicks idea can cause some to miss symptoms of preterm labor.

    Williams. "Maternal Adaptation to Pregnancy." Ch. 8, p. 210.

MYTH #38: Women are more likely to go into labor during a full moon.

1. Danish study.

    Trap, R., Helm, P., Lidegaard, O., Helm, E. "Premature rupture of the Fetal Membranes, the Phases of the Moon and Barometric Readings." *Gynecologic and Obstetric Investigation.* 28:14–18. 1989.
2. Mozambique study.

Strolego, F., Gigli, C., Bugalho, A. "The Influence of Lunar Phases on the Frequency of Deliveries." *Minerva Ginecologica.* 43:359–63. 1991. Author's note: Abstract only. (It was the only portion translated into English. The paper itself was written in Italian.)

3. French Study.

Guillon, P., Guillon, D., Lansaac, J., Soutoul, J.H., Bertrand, P., Hornecker, J.P. "Births, Fertility, Rhythms and Lunar Cycle: a Statistical Study of 5,927,978 Births." *Journal de Gynecologie, Obsetrique et Biologie de la Reproduction.* 15:265–71. 1986. Author's note: Abstract only. (It was the only portion translated into English. The paper itself was written in French.)

MYTH #39: Pregnant women are more likely to break their bag of waters during storms.

1. Danish study (also cited above in reference on full moon).

Trap, R., Helm, P., Lidegaard, O., Helm, E. "Premature Rupture of the Fetal Membranes, the Phases of the Moon and Barometer Readings." *Gynecologic and Obstetric Investigations.* 28:14–8. 1989.

MYTH #41: The doctor can predict when labor will start by means of a cervical exam near the end of pregnancy.

1. The Bishop score.

Friedman, E.A. *Labor: Clinical Evaluation and Management.* 2nd edition. East Norwalk, Connecticut: Appleton-Century-Crofts, 1978.

2. The relationship between cervical dilation and preterm labor.

Williams. "Preterm and Postterm Pregnancy and Fetal Growth Retardation." Ch. 38, p. 866.

MYTH #42: First-time mothers tend to deliver late and second-time mothers tend to deliver early (or vice versa).

1. The studies regarding the due date.
   Williams. "Prenatal Care." Ch. 9, p. 249.
2. Swedish study.
   Bergsjo, P., Denman, III, D.W., Hoffman, H.J., Meirik, O. "Duration of Human Singleton Pregnancy: A Population-based Study." *Acta Obstet. Gynecol. Scand.* 69:197–207. 1990.

MYTH #43: I should donate blood before delivery.

1. Low rate of transfusion during delivery.
   Sherman, S.J., Geenspoon, J.S., Nelson, J.M., Paul, R.H. "Obstetric Hemorrhage and Blood Utilization." *Journal of Reproductive Medicine.* 38:929–34. 1993.
2. Skeptical view of auto-donation.
   Andres, R.L., Piacquadio, K.M., Resnik, R. "A Reappraisal of the Need for Autologous Blood Donation in the Obstetric Patient." *American Journal of Obstetrics and Gynecology.* 163:1551–3. 1990.

MYTH #44: My family should donate blood for me before delivery.

1. German paper regarding higher risk in designated donor blood.
   Timoteo, R., Grunenberg, R., Bloedorn, H., Kruger, J. "Comparison of the Suitability of First Time and Related Blood Donors." *Beitrage zur Infusionstherapie.* 26:267–9. 1990. Author's note: Abstract in English only. The paper itself was originally written in German.

CHAPTER FOUR
Childbirth

The Amniotic Membranes

MYTH #45: A "dry" birth is dangerous.

1. Premature rupture of the membranes occurs 10 percent of the time.

   Creasy and Resnik. Garite, T.J. "Premature Rupture of the Membranes." Ch. 41, p. 625.

MYTH #46: A woman who has ruptured membranes before the onset of labor in a previous labor is likely to do so in subsequent births.

1. Incidence at term.

   Creasy and Resnik. Garite, T.J. "Premature Rupture of the Membranes." Ch. 41, p. 625.

2. Incidence before term.

   Williams. "Preterm and Posterm Pregnancy and Fetal Growth Retardation. Ch. 38, p. 862.

3. Relationship of preterm PROM to preterm PROM in subsequent pregnancies.

   Creasy and Resnik. Garite TJ. "Premature Rupture of the Membranes." Ch. 41, p. 626.

   Ekwo, E.E., Gosselink, C.A., Moawad, A. "Unfavorable Outcome in Penultimate Pregnancy and Premature Rupture of Membranes in Successive Pregnancy." *Obstetrics and Gynecology.* 80:166–72. 1992.

4. Relationship of term PROM to term PROM in subsequent pregnancies.

   Gosselink, C.A., Ekwo, E.E., Woolson, R.F., Moawad, A.,

Long, C.R. "Dietary Habits, Pregnancy Weight, and Weight Gain During Pregnancy: Risk of Preterm Rupture of Amniotic Sac Membranes." *Acta Obstet Gynecol Scand.* 71:425–38. 1992.

Pain Relief in Labor

MYTH #48: A common complication of epidural anesthesia is paralysis.

1. Cited safety statistics for anesthesia.
   Philip, B.K. "Complications of Regional Anesthesia." Ch. 14, p. 287. In: Ostheimer, Gerard W. *Manual of Obstetric Anesthesia.* New York: Churchill Livingstone, 1984.
2. Death rate from auto accidents.
   Hatcher, R.A., Trussel, J., Stewart, F., et.al. *Contraceptive Technology.* 16th revised edition. New York: Irvington Publishers, Inc., 1994, p. 125.

Labor

MYTH #54: Walking tends to help the progress of labor.

1. Discussion of studies regarding ambulation.
   Smith, M.A., Ruffin, M.T., Green, L.A. "The Rational Management of Labor." *American Family Physician.* 47:1471–81. 1993.

MYTH #55: Healing from a tear is less painful than healing from an episiotomy (or vice versa).

1. Study comparing pain after childbirth laceration versus pain after episiotomy.

    Abraham, S., Child, A., Ferry, J., Vizzard, J., Mira, M. "Recovery after Childbirth: a Preliminary Prospective Study." *Medical Journal of Australia.* 152:9–12. 1990.

Delivery

MYTH #57: Vacuum and forceps deliveries are dangerous and should always be avoided.

1. Safety of operative delivery.

    Creasy and Resnik. Bowes, Jr., W.A. "Clinical Aspects of Normal and Abnormal Labor." Ch. 35, p. 548–9.

Cesarean Delivery

MYTH #58: Fetal distress is the most common reason for Cesarean birth.

1. Reasons for Cesarean, by frequency.

    Williams. "Cesarean Section and Cesarean Hysterectomy." Ch. 26, p. 593–4.

MYTH #59: A woman who has a history of genital herpes will require Cesarean delivery.

1. Cesarean section appropriate only for visible lesions.
2. Incidence of neonatal herpes.
3. Majority of neonates afflicted with Herpes are born to mothers without lesions.

"Perinatal Herpes Simplex Virus Infections." *ACOG Technical Bulletin.* No. 122, November 1988.

4. Only 2 to 5% who have HSV will have outbreak close to labor.

Hensleigh, P.A. "Herpes in Pregnancy—It's Especially Serious for Neonate." *Contemporary Ob/Gyn.* October 1994, pp. 25–40.

5. Maternal mortality rate.

Williams. "Obstetrics in a Broad Perspective." Ch. 1, p. 3.

CHAPTER FIVE:
The Baby Before, During, and After Birth

Gender Prediction

MYTH #60: The fetal heart rate provides a clue about gender.

1. Obstetricians cannot accurately measure the rate.

Hon, E.H. "The electronic evaluation of the fetal heart rate." *American Journal of Obstetrics and Gynecology.* 75:1215. 1958.

2. Book on fetal monitoring:

Freeman, R.K., Garite, T.J., Nageotte, M.P. *Fetal Heart Rate Monitoring. 2nd edition.* Baltimore: Williams & Wilkins, 1991.

MYTH #64: Having sex before ovulation increase the chance of a boy.

1. Increased chance of having a boy from coitus before pregnancy.

Gray, R.H. "Natural Family Planning and Sex Selection: Fact or Fiction?" *American Journal of Obstetrics and Gynecology.* 165:1982–4. 1991.

World Health Organization. "A Prospective Multicentre Study of the Ovulation Method of Natural Family Planning. IV. The Outcome of Pregnancy." *Fertility and Sterility.* 41:593–8. 1984.

2. Increased chance of miscarriage and birth defects.

Gray, R.H. and Kambic, R.T. "Epidemiological Studies of Natural Family Planning." *Human Reproduction.* 3:693–8. 1988.

Simpson, J.L., Gray, R.H., Queenan, J.T., et al. "Fetal Outcome Among Pregnancies in Natural Family Planning Acceptors: An International Cohort Study." *American Journal of Obstetrics and Gynecology.* 165:1981–2. 1991.

Fetal Health

MYTH #66: Having the umbilical cord wound around the baby's neck is a major cause of newborn death and injury.

1. One-fourth of live-born babies have the cord around the neck.

   Williams. "Conduct of Normal Labor and Delivery." Ch. 34, p. 381.

MYTH #69: Streptococcus is a particularly dangerous bacteria and is a common cause of newborn injury and death.

1. All statistics and recommendations.

   GBS infections in pregnancy. *ACOG Technical Bulletin.* No. 170. July 1992.

Birth Defects

Myth #70: A normal ultrasound excludes birth defects.

1. Rate of false negative scans in fetuses subsequently shown to have heart defects.
   Williams. "Ultrasound in Obstetrics." Ch. 46, p. 1050.

Myth #71: A leading cause of mental retardation is lack of oxygen during labor.

1. Rate of mental retardation in population.
   Freeman, R.K., Garite, T.J., Nageotte, M.P. *Fetal Heart Rate Monitoring. 2nd edition.* Baltimore: Williams and Wilkins, 1991, pp. 21–5.
2. Estimated contribution of labor problems to mental retardation.
   Williams. "Diseases and Injuries of the Fetus and Newborn Infant." Ch. 44, p. 1002.

Myth #72: A leading cause of cerebral palsy is lack of oxygen during labor.

"Fetal and Neonatal Neurologic Injury." *ACOG Technical Bulletin.* No. 163. January 1992.

Myth #73: Medical X rays pose a significant threat to the fetus and should always be avoided.

1. All factual information.
   Williams. "Imaging Modalities During Pregnancy." Ch. 43, pp. 981–5.

CHAPTER SIX:
Post-Partum

Recovery

MYTH #74: Childbirth scars are a common cause of painful intercourse long after the birth.

1. Cited study.
   Abraham, S., Child, A., Ferry, J., Vizzard, J., Mira, M. "Recovery after Childbirth: a Preliminary Prospective Study." *Medical Journal of Australia.* 152:9–12. 1990.

MYTH #76: Postpartum "blues" are widely experienced after delivery and are often severe and long lasting.

1. Symptoms.
   Sciarra. O'Hara, M.W. "Postpartum Mental Disorders." Vol. 6, Ch. 84, p. 1.
2. Incidence.
   Sciarra. O'Hara, M.W. "Postpartum Mental Disorders." Vol. 6, Ch. 84, p. 3.
3. Causes.
   Williams. "The Puerperium." Ch. 18, p. 469.

MYTH #77: Women with postpartum depression will make bad mothers because they really do not want their babies.

1. Incidence.
   Sciarra. O'Hara, M.W. "Postpartum Mental Disorders." Vol. 6, Ch. 84, p. 3.
   Williams. "The Puerperium." Ch. 18, p. 469.
2. Background incidence of depression in the general population.

Sciarra. O'Hara, M.W. "Postpartum Mental Disorders." Vol. 6, Ch. 84, p. 3.

Nursing

MYTH #78: Mothers who nurse cannot get pregnant.

1. Facts about lactation and fertility.
   Hatcher, et. al. *Contraceptive Technology, 16th edition.* New York: Irvington Publishers, Inc., 1994, p. 435.

BIRTH
DAY!

PREFACE

Despite the vast amount of reading matter available on pregnancy, there is still very little written for expectant mothers about the vital facts of actually having a baby. Adequate information about the language of birth and the actual medical process a woman in labor faces is simply not available. As the end of the pregnancy draws near and as you, an expectant mother, become more uncomfortable and anxious, you will find peace of mind in knowledge of the birth process.

When you enter the hospital to give birth, your level of anxiety or stage of labor might not permit extended discussion with your doctor or nurses. My goal in this book is to cover most of the possible medical interventions commonly used during childbirth, so that you will be informed and prepared as labor progresses. This means providing you with a better understanding not only of the physiological changes of labor, but also of the medical choices available and the reasons for your doctor's actions. In a society of growing complexity, there is commonly a gap between scientific advancements and a person's ability to cope as a patient. Today, there are numerous diagnostic procedures and tests along with a broad array of medications to help with the comfort and safety of childbirth. With the information and perspective provided here, I hope to make the medical technology of hospital childbirth less strange and confusing.

In the following chapters, you will find answers to question such as: When is the normal time for my water bag to break? Why do doctors sometimes break it, and is that a safe practice? What risks do pain medications pose for my baby? What is false labor? How do doctors and nurses monitor the health of the baby during labor? Why do doctors do episiotomies? What are the risks of cesarean section, and why are the rates rising in this country? Being familiar with the many aspects of labor and delivery will help you to have a good birth experience. Childbirth in a modern hospital is not a frightening experience, especially if you know what to expect during the twelve to twenty-four hours before you give birth.

When I first gave thought to writing a book on childbirth, I was impressed by the general lack of information available. This gap was especially surprising given the sheer quantity of books on the subject of pregnancy. What I discovered was that most of these books are too general and spend little time on the most anxiety-provoking moments of pregnancy—the actual "birth day." With this book, I have tried to educate mothers-to-be about the many facts an obstetrician considers when making a recommendation for testing or treating a laboring patient. My experience has been that an educated patient is able to make an informed decision about medical choices as they arise, while an unprepared patient may decline a medical intervention because it carries with it some measurable though small risk, even though in doing so she places herself or her baby at a disadvantage. What I hope you will learn in reading this book is that not only do all procedures carry varying degrees of risks and benefits, but also that taking no action at all may also carry risks.

Increased knowledge about labor and childbirth should lead to a greater sense of trust between you and your doctor, and to a better level of communication. It may also guide your choice in the event that your physician asks for your preference concerning different methods of treatment. Bear in mind that, as a doctor, I view my role as an adviser and educator, *not* a decision maker. Many doctors in the 1990's share this view, and we look to our patients either to decide among treatment options or to make clear their preferences. It may surprise some readers to know that an occasional patient will be distressed with this philosophy. "You're the doctor. You should know," they will tell me. While it is true that I do have more knowledge and experience about health-related issues than my patients, many decisions in medicine are subjective and not that different from choosing a favorite color. To continue this metaphor, I am content to describe the "colors" and let the patient pick. If asked, I certainly can make the choice, but I would normally expect the patient to choose. This concept is fundamental to the doctor-patient relationship: Am I merely the adviser, or am I the decision maker? Most doctors, myself included, feel comfortable in either role, but the point is that you, the expectant mother, should know in your mind which style of doctoring you prefer. This book will be particularly helpful for women who wish to retain control over the decision-making process. It is intended to provide a foundation of facts and familiarize you sufficiently with medical interventions so that you feel comfortable choosing different options when they are offered. In the vast majority of labors, both mother and baby come out just fine without any need for medical intervention. I view my role as providing emotional support, first and foremost, then providing pain relief if requested, and, finally, intervening only in those rare circumstances where health or safety are threatened.

On a personal note, and as an obstetrician who has delivered babies for many years, I still find each birth miraculous and special. As a father of three, I can say that the joy of bringing new life into the world is unique and surpasses any of my other experiences. The very decision to become a parent always carries the risk that things may not turn out as we hope, but the rewards can be no greater. Congratulations on your adventure, and good luck.

Chapter One

WHEN WILL MY BABY ARRIVE?

You may be convinced that your obstetrician has some secret insight into when you will go into labor. No such predictive power exists. On the other hand, predicting your baby's arrival is not nearly as uncertain as betting on a horse race. Unlike picking winners at the track, medical science has some sound ways of bracketing the time of your baby's arrival.

WHAT DOES MY DUE DATE MEAN?

The date on which the baby is due is obviously of keen interest to you. This is the deadline for the end of your long and uncomfortable pregnancy. Should you cancel plans for that day and simply pencil in "hospital" on your calendar? Don't do it. Less than 10 percent of women deliver on their due date. Roughly half of them deliver before this date, and the remainder deliver afterward.

How is the due date assigned? It is generally calculated to be forty weeks after the first day of your last menstrual period. This assumes that you have had regular menstrual periods about every

1

twenty-eight days, and that you had no vaginal bleeding after your last period. Implicit in this calculation is the assumption that you ovulated (and conceived) roughly two weeks after the beginning of your menstrual period. In women who have just stopped using birth control pills or who have had irregular cycles, such calculations tend to be less accurate because the timing of ovulation is less predictable.

Why is the due date calculated from the first day of the last period rather than from conception? After all, conception takes place at about the time of ovulation—not during the period. Historically, the notion of ovulation, or the production and discharge of the eggs from an ovarian follicle, is a relatively new idea. For thousands of years mothers-to-be and doctors have been calculating that pregnancy began when the period stopped. As a result, the due date and all references to gestational age in medical texts and reports of ultrasound pictures use the forty-week determination from the start of the period, which is after an elapse of nine months and one week.

This may bring on some confusion about how to convert your obstetrician's "weeks" to everyone else's "months." It is true that a pregnancy lasts for nine months, but these are calendar months— almost all with more than twenty-eight days. Thus, the pregnancy lasts for approximately forty weeks, not thirty-six weeks. When someone asks "How far along are you?" it is easier to understand the answer "I am in the seventh month," however approximate, than it is to figure out "I am in the twenty-seventh week."

Many of my patients have their own way of calculating their due dates. I will never forget one mother, pregnant with her fourth baby, who brushed aside science and medical experience with her own crystal ball forecast. And she proved to be right! At each prenatal visit, she announced that she would deliver on "Thursday the nineteenth," which was in her thirty-sixth week of pregnancy. Each time she came into my office I patiently explained that a precise birth date was impossible to predict so far in advance and that the date she predicted was actually preterm.

"Delivery at this time would pose a small threat of prematurity to the baby," I intoned. Well, of course, she went into labor on

'Thursday the nineteenth. The baby was born after only one hour of contractions. The woman, looking up at me with a happy grin, proclaimed, "I told you so." For the betterment of science, I had to ask her how she knew. "Why, Dr. Benson, it was obvious. My first baby was born on Monday the seventh, my second on Tuesday the eleventh, and the third was on Wednesday the thirteenth. I knew my fourth would be born on a Thursday that fell on the nineteenth of the month, because that date was a prime number greater than thirteen." I was thankful that Thursday the nineteenth was not in her sixth month.

The accuracy of your projected due date can be confirmed by examining the size of your uterus during prenatal visits. If there seems to be a large difference between the actual size and the expected size, an ultrasound picture can be obtained to measure your fetus. The accuracy of an ultrasound in predicting the due date depends on the number and timing of the studies. For instance, a single ultrasound obtained in the third trimester is almost useless in assigning a due date since the sizes of babies this late in gestation are so variable. In general, ultrasounds in the first two trimesters are reasonably accurate in establishing a due date but they are not inherently more accurate than making a prediction based on the date of the last menstrual period. In my practice, we do not change the due date assigned by menstrual dating unless the ultrasound suggests that the fetus is more than one week younger or older than we would have suspected by menstrual dating alone. Even with a due date based on accurate assumptions, a woman is likely to deliver on some other day.

What does the word "term" mean? The baby is term if it is delivered in a four-week period centered on the due date—from thirty-eight weeks to forty-two weeks gestation. This is the ideal time frame for the baby's arrival. Babies born before thirty-eight weeks are preterm, or premature. After forty-two weeks, they are postterm. Problems can arise at either extreme, although this affects only a relatively small number of women—roughly 5 percent of pregnancies will end prematurely and another 5 percent will last too long. You are not really overdue from a medical point of view until you are a full two weeks past the due date.

So when will my baby arrive? By thirty-six weeks, you will be looking for any clue that will help pin down the delivery date. Perhaps your vaginal discharge has increased, your occasional contractions are stronger, or your friends tell you the baby has dropped. None of these observations has great value in predicting the big day. Doctors are not immune from this guessing game either. We like to project how busy our coming days and nights will be. Four weeks before your due date, your doctor may start weekly cervical checks to confirm that the baby's head is coming first and to determine the dilation of the cervix. Typically your cervix thins, softens, and dilates slightly as your due date approaches. As a rule, the more dilated the cervix is, the more likely you are to go into labor in the near future.

Pregnant women are so unpredictable that this dilation rule may not be very helpful in guessing when you will deliver. I remember a patient who was four centimeters dilated at thirty-two weeks. We gave her antilabor medication to prevent a premature birth. I made a small wager with my partner that she would deliver before thirty-six weeks. My partner bet she would deliver later. The patient delivered a day before her due date—a full eight weeks after our initial assessment. Such unpredictability works both ways. I also had a patient who was eager to deliver two weeks before her due date but was not dilated at all. After hesitating with the bad news, I told her that I did not think she would deliver within the next two weeks. She had the baby that night.

WHEN SHOULD I CALL MY DOCTOR?

The answer to this question is highly variable. Some doctors prefer to be called before you go to the hospital; others prefer to be notified by the nurses after you have been examined and are settled in. Occasionally, doctors will suggest that you call the labor and delivery suite directly for some of the more routine questions such as, "Am I in labor?" Your doctor will make his or her preference known as your due date approaches, but be sure to ask if you are uncertain. There are other circumstances when you should call your doctor. One such normal occurrence is when the bag of waters breaks, with or without accompanying contractions. Some physicians prefer to have you go directly to the hospital; others will have you wait at home until the onset of strong, regular contractions (see also Chapter Four).

Your doctor should always be made aware of abnormal conditions you may be experiencing. These include severe, unremitting abdominal pain, heavy vaginal bleeding without mucus (see mucus plug in Chapter Three), and abdominal cramping or contractions that occur four times or more in an hour if the due date is more than two weeks distant. Also, you should talk with your doctor more often than weekly if you have special conditions known in advance of labor such as breech or twin gestation. Whenever you are uncertain about the conditions under which you should notify your obstetrician, you should call to ask.

A good guideline to use in calling your doctor is that if anxiety over a given issue is distracting you or keeping you awake, you should call—even at night or on a weekend. Often enough, a short explanation over the phone by your physician can ease your mind. Obstetricians know they have a twenty-four-hour-a-day, seven-day-a-week job.

Although we expect to be called at any time of the day or night, many patients try to be considerate and not bother us at night. While it's true that prescription refills are best handled during office hours, many pregnant patients seem reluctant to call for things that genuinely require attention. As doctors, we often worry more about those patients whom we suspect won't call even if they have a genuine problem.

CALL FOR

1. Ruptured membranes.
2. Contractions every five minutes (first baby) or every ten minutes for one hour (second baby and beyond).
3. Heavy vaginal bleeding, severe pain, greatly decreased fetal movement.
4. Anxiety or questions keeping you awake.

WHEN DO I GO TO THE HOSPITAL?

There are two reasons for you to labor in a hospital: access to pain relief and safety. Each is a separate consideration.

Most doctors prefer to avoid giving narcotics or an epidural (see Chapters Nine and Ten) until it is clear that you are progressing well in labor. If narcotics are given too early, they tend to become less effective in subsequent doses. Both narcotics and an epidural anesthetic can slow labor at least momentarily if given too soon. Although this slowing is often only temporary and can be counteracted by giving a labor-inducing medication called oxytocin (Pitocin), most obstetricians find such tampering with nature to be undesirable. As a result, it is common practice for your doctor to withhold medication until you are clearly dilating.

I am often asked, "How dilated do I have to be before you will give me something for pain?" This is a difficult question to answer when it is phrased this way. Labor is defined as contractions that result in cervical dilation—not just contractions by themselves. You can still be quite uncomfortable with "early" contractions before you begin to dilate. The amount of dilation is less important than whether or not dilation is taking place. Most obstetricians do not have a minimum dilation before they consider prescribing pain medication or epidurals. We prefer to individualize. Also, your doctor will often prescribe medication if you are terribly uncomfortable even if you are not dilating. The decision to have pain medication is yours, since only you can know how much pain you are experiencing. Rarely will your doctor not give you pain medication, and that would be because of safety concerns.

What about arriving at the hospital in time to assure the safest course of labor for both you and your baby? In a normal pregnancy without medical problems such as diabetes, high blood pressure, or a compromised fetus, the later stages of labor are the most important time to monitor both of you. From the point of view of safety and comfort, it is desirable to arrive at the hospital when the cervix begins to dilate steadily.

How can you tell when your cervix begins to dilate? Without pelvic exams over time, you and your doctor can only guess. However, there are some useful guidelines that apply for most women. These clues are different for women with their first baby and those in subsequent labors. Remember that these are general principles; your doctor may wish to modify them depending on your particular situation.

If this is your first baby, remember that contractions that result in cervical dilation must grow stronger, come closer together, and persist for several hours. If the contractions are not steadily getting stronger over time, or if they come at irregular intervals, cervical dilation is doubtful. Also, good labor contractions are so strong that you would not usually think of them as strong menstrual cramps. When you undergo labor with your first child and are actively dilating, you will not be inclined to smile or talk during these contractions. Ordinarily, after one to two hours of strong contractions that last for more than forty-five seconds and come at least every five minutes, you should contact your doctor or proceed to the hospital, depending on your obstetrician's instructions.

Advice for mothers in labor with second and subsequent babies is different. Since these labors tend to be faster and more unpredictable, you should contact your doctor after only an hour of regular, strong contractions that occur every ten minutes or less.

Though these directions may make sense during a calm moment, the onset of labor is always anxiety-provoking. Even obstetricians can get upset. With my wife's most recent pregnancy, she had contractions for brief stretches of time. Every time she held her abdomen or paused during an activity, I stopped what I was doing to ask if she was having a contraction. This got her rattled. The last days of pregnancy are ones of apprehensive waiting—even for the father who specializes in obstetrics.

It is always helpful to know the route to the hospital and to practice driving it once or twice in advance. You need to know where to enter the hospital after hours or on weekends. Even with a new maternity wing at the hospital where I practice, the entrance at night is still through the emergency room. There are plenty of stories about panicky fathers-to-be rushing from locked door to locked door. You should not assume that the delivery will take place during normal working hours when there are medical personnel readily available to direct you to the right entrance.

WHAT HAPPENS IF MY BABY DOES NOT WAIT UNTIL I ARRIVE AT THE HOSPITAL?

Although this is a frightening experience, there are three key points to keep in mind. First, having your baby before arriving at the hospital is very unusual. Second, one of the chief reasons for delivering in a hospital is access to pain relief. If the labor is so quick that your baby delivers before arrival at the hospital, obviously pain relief is less urgently needed. Third, fast deliveries tend to occur in healthy, uncomplicated pregnancies. Under these circumstances, you and your baby are often the least likely to need medical intervention. Your baby has to fit easily through the birth canal to deliver so readily, and you will not be exhausted from a long labor. If you experience precipitous birth, you can consider yourself lucky, although you may not realize this right away.

Birth can usually be expected within minutes when the baby begins to crown. This means that the baby's scalp hair is visible to another observer at your vaginal opening between contractions and that the birth canal bulges outward from the pressure of the head as the baby descends. If you are alone, you probably cannot see the opening of the birth canal, but you would feel a great deal of pressure near your rectum a few minutes before the birth. For your first baby, birth may still be ten to thirty minutes away. Again, delivery before arrival at the hospital is nearly unheard of with a first labor at term. With subsequent labors, birth can occur sooner—within one to two minutes of crowning. At this advanced stage of labor, you will usually be grunting involuntarily due to the natural reflex to push the baby out.

If it is obvious that the baby is likely to arrive before your arrival at the hospital, STOP THE CAR. Do not drive recklessly in an effort to arrive before the baby is born. Serious traffic accidents have been known to occur in a headlong rush to the hospital. The instructions below have been written assuming that you are driving with your husband, a relative, or friend. If possible, avoid driving by yourself, although these instructions can be carried out all by yourself. When it is clear that birth is imminent (i.e., when you are crowning with a second or subsequent pregnancy), do the following:

1. Stop the car and pull off the road to a safe location.
2. Move to a flat surface, such as the ground next to the car. In the event that the weather is very cold, however, it may be better to stay in the car, keeping as flat as possible.
3. To accomplish the birth, you should push down for ten seconds at a time with the contractions. Hold your breath and tighten your abdominal muscles as though you were having a bowel movement. As the baby's head emerges, it should be supported gently until the shoulders are delivered. If you are alone, you cannot support the baby's head and should simply push to deliver the shoulders. The baby is very slippery and will slide out very quickly once the shoulders are out. Be sure that you are on a flat surface and that the baby does not have a great distance to drop from the vaginal opening to the ground. If there is a delay of more than a full minute in delivery of the shoulders, the baby's head can be *gently* directed downward to guide the front shoulder under the pubic bone. If you are alone, simply push down on your lower abdomen just above the pubic bone.
4. Once the baby is out, there can be a delay of several seconds to a minute before he takes his first gasp. Tickle his feet or scratch his back to let him know he has been born.
5. Once the newborn makes breathing noises or begins to cry, dry him off thoroughly and keep him covered in dry clothing. A newborn can get cold quickly, particularly if wet.
6. At this point the baby will still be attached to the umbilical cord. Generally there will be a substantial gush of blood just before the placenta delivers. If the placenta does not deliver within five minutes, proceed to the hospital with the baby

still attached to the cord (and to mom). If the placenta is expelled before arrival at the hospital, your abdomen should be firmly massaged just below the umbilicus (belly button). This will be uncomfortable, but it will help your uterus contract and thus cut down on blood loss.

7. It is not necessary for you to cut the umbilical cord before arriving at the hospital. After several minutes the cord seals off naturally. This occurs when the cord stops pulsating. If, for some reason, the cord needs to be cut, wait until it stops beating, then firmly tie a string around it about six inches away from the baby's abdominal wall. Cut the cord with a clean, though not necessarily sterile, instrument on the side of the string away from the baby. Blood will leak out of that portion of the cord that has been separated from the baby.

Delivering a baby is an inherently bloody event and is associated with some pain. On average, mothers lose roughly one pint of blood during the birth. This can seem like quite a bit even though most mothers are no worse for it. If nothing else, think of the exciting story you'll be able to tell your child about his or her dramatic entrance!

WHAT IS "FALSE" LABOR?

So-called false labor can cause much anxiety. Often, as the contractions wax and wane over the hours, you will agonize over whether or not you should go to the hospital. The term false labor is a misnomer, since the contractions are certainly real and can be very uncomfortable. A better term for contractions that do not lead to progressive cervical dilation over several hours is prodromal labor. Particularly with a first pregnancy, there may be very noticeable preparatory periods in which relatively strong contractions occur frequently and then subside after several hours. You can think of this as the uterus warming up for labor. Prodromal labor can be difficult to distinguish from the labor that leads to cervical dilation. Indeed, sometimes the only way to tell the difference is for you to go to the hospital or your doctor's office for a cervical exam. There is no shame in getting examined and then returning home, if appropriate. As a rule, the contractions that lead to cervical change persist for hours and get stronger. They also tend to be regularly spaced and to be separated by at least one to two minutes.

This uncomfortable prodromal labor can last for twenty-four hours or even for days, although it rarely does. You may be too uncomfortable to sleep and can become exhausted, even before the onset of more active labor. Obstetricians will occasionally intervene in this prolonged prodromal labor, lessening the discomfort with narcotic sedation or medication (Pitocin) to induce contractions so that you go into labor. Our recommendations depend on the particular circumstances of the pregnancy and your wishes. If you choose a sound night's sleep with medication, you will generally wake up in either a good labor pattern or with the contractions greatly reduced.

WHAT DO I DO IF MY BABY STOPS MOVING?

There is a persistent myth among pregnant women that the fetal movements decrease just before the onset of labor. This is not true. No doubt you know that lack of movement is significant, but your baby's movements are so variable from hour to hour and day to day that the situation can be difficult to assess. Movements within the womb can be an important sign of your baby's health, and a large decrease in movement may indicate a baby in jeopardy. Although very few babies sicken within the uterus during pregnancy, paying attention to fetal movements is such an easy thing to do that you should be aware of them. You should call your obstetrician if you feel no movement in a twelve-hour period or if you notice significantly decreased movement in a twenty-four-hour period.

If you do not wish to wait a full day, you can still get a good picture of your baby's status by following these steps:

1. Count your baby's movements from the time you wake up in the morning.

2. Each and every type of movement counts as one movement, whether it's a kick, a punch, or a roll.

3. After you count ten movements, you're through monitoring for the day. The baby is fine if you can count at least ten movements in an eight-hour period.

4. If you have not counted ten movements by 4:00 P.M., you should lie down on either side for sixty minutes and monitor the movements more carefully. You can be distracted by other things during the day and sometimes miss the movements of even an active fetus.

5. If your baby does not move at least twice during this hour, you should call your doctor. Babies can show highly variable movement patterns from day to day and hour to hour. In my own experience as an obstetrician, I cannot recall a single time when one of my patients noticed decreased movements and her baby was ill. However, I always monitor the fetal pulse if a woman is concerned that her baby has become less active.

These recommendations are designed to help you become more aware of the your baby's patterns of activity. What if your baby does have decreased movement in a given day? Your doctor will have you come to the office or hospital to get a test called a nonstress test, or an NST. This is a painless, thirty-minute test during which a special ultrasound microphone is placed on your abdomen to register the baby's pulse over time. A separate sensor is placed on your abdomen to detect contractions (see Chapter Four on contraction monitoring). The vast majority of mothers and their babies pass this test with flying colors and can go about their business. Very rarely additional testing may be needed.

Some patients say they feel foolish for bothering their doctor when they feel decreased movement. Often enough, the baby becomes much more active on the way to the hospital or office. Just the same, we are happy to be called and to find that the fetus is moving normally. Reassurance is one of the most important services your doctor can provide. Do not hesitate to ask.

Chapter Two

LABOR

Contractions should be more bearable if you have an understanding of what to expect before labor begins. What is labor? When does it start? When will it end?

WHAT IS LABOR?

Many people think that labor is synonymous with contractions. This explains the horror stories told about unfortunate women "in labor" for three days or a week. The correct obstetrical definition of labor is "progressive cervical effacement and dilation in the face of regular uterine contractions." While it is true that a woman must be contracting to be considered in labor, she must also simultaneously experience opening of the cervix, or tip of the womb.

Determination of labor can be difficult even for the experts. More often than not, we have to observe you in the maternity ward for a few hours and do a series of exams of your cervix before we can be sure it is actually dilating. Talking with you on the phone about your contractions can help us guess about what is going on, but there is no substitute for a check of the cervix.

HOW DOES MY CERVIX DILATE?

How does the tip of the womb open during labor? Although the biochemical aspects of labor are not well understood, the dilation process itself is predictable over time and easily describable. When you are not in labor your cervix is a cylinder of tissue approximately one- to two-inches long and one inch in diameter. The cylinder has a small canal running through its length, permitting sperm to enter the uterus from the vagina and, conversely, allowing menstrual blood to pass out of the uterus into the vagina. This canal is normally small enough to prevent the passage of a cotton swab into the uterus. Even so, its opening is visible to your doctor and is known as the cervical os, or opening.

You can actually feel your own cervix. It is a bump deep within the vagina that has the consistency of the end of your nose. The opening of the canal can be felt as a small indentation. Toward the end of pregnancy the cervix becomes quite difficult to feel on your own due to the changing position of the fetus. You cannot reliably check your own dilation in the third trimester and should not attempt to do so.

The baby must pass through the cervix to be born. The widest part of your baby is the head, which is usually about ten centimeters (approximately four inches) in diameter. Therefore, the cervix must dilate, or open, to ten centimeters by the end of labor. This point, when reached, is also known as completely dilated.

In measuring the progress of labor, the nurse or physician will check you for three things on pelvic examination: dilation, effacement, and station. As mentioned, dilation varies from closed to ten centimeters. Cervical effacement refers to cervical thickness and is measured as a percentage. A completely effaced (100 percent) cervix is paper-thin. Although dilation and effacement measure different aspects of the cervix, they are related in that the cervix tends to thin out as it opens. Effacement is typically, but not always, completed by the time the cervix is four centimeters dilated. As a result, observing the change in cervical effacement is most useful for measuring your labor progress in the early stages.

Station refers to the location of the lowest portion of your baby within your pelvis. Zero station means that the widest part of the baby's head has entered your pelvic inlet. This station is also called engaged. The baby is assigned a minus station if the head is above zero station and a plus station if the head has descended beyond this point. As labor progresses, the cervix thins and dilates, and the head descends through the birth canal.

All this special medical jargon was not originally meant to communicate with you but was developed to describe precisely the current delivery status to the medical personnel involved. Doctors are happy to report to you on your dilation and effacement. As always, you should feel free to ask questions.

HOW LONG WILL I BE IN LABOR?

Obstetricians divide labor into three stages. The first is by far the longest and ends with complete dilation of the cervix. The second stage is the time from complete dilation to the delivery of the infant. The third stage ends with the delivery of the placenta, or afterbirth. Your subsequent labors will usually be shorter and easier than your first labor.

STAGES OF LABOR

FIRST: Start of dilation to complete dilation of the cervix
  Latent phase: Slow dilation (generally ends at four centimeters)
  Active phase: Rapid dilation (generally four centimeters to ten centimeters)
SECOND: From complete dilation to birth (pushing occurs)
THIRD: From birth to delivery of the placenta

There are several important features to be aware of even before your first labor begins. Usually your baby's head will drop in the pelvis several days to several weeks before the onset of labor. You might notice this drop as you feel the baby lower in your body close to term, although you will not always be aware of this change in position. As a result of this drop, it is common to begin your first labor with the baby's head at, or close to, zero station. Also, your cervix begins to thin and dilate in the weeks before labor, but you will often begin your first labor at two centimeters or less dilation. In contrast, with your subsequent labors you will usually not notice the baby dropping within the pelvis until just before or even during labor. It is not unusual to begin labor at three or four centimeters dilated.

The First Stage: Latent Phase (First Labor)

The early part of labor is known as the latent phase, although the contractions are quite noticeable and hardly latent. Your first regular contractions will probably feel like strong menstrual cramps and begin about twenty minutes apart. These early contractions often last for only thirty seconds. Over a period of hours, the contractions gradually get stronger and occur more frequently. At this point you are usually still able to talk during a contraction. The cervix typically does not begin to thin or dilate significantly until you have experienced contractions for several hours. By this time, contractions occur at least as frequently as every five minutes and last for more than forty-five seconds. You might be distracted by the strength of these contractions, but you are unlikely to want pain medication. During this first part of labor you can pass time by walking around or taking a shower. The contractions are noticeable enough to interfere with normal activity such as sleeping or work but are usually not so uncomfortable that you would want to go to the hospital.

You may take as long as twenty hours to go from "long and closed" to four centimeters dilated in the presence of regular, frequent contractions. Though this may seem like a long time, there are three facts that should make this period easier for you to live with. First, you usually do not begin even your first labor completely long and closed. As mentioned above, women at term usually have at least some thinning of the cervix before the beginning of labor. Second, for much of this time the regular, frequent contractions are not as strong as in later labor and are generally quite tolerable, although they will probably prevent sleep or other normal activity. Finally, you are likely to dilate more quickly than the minimum 0.2 centimeters per hour.

The First Stage: Active Phase (First Labor)

Your active phase of labor, or the period of more rapid cervical dilation, usually begins between two to four centimeters. By this time your contractions have become closer and stronger until they occur every three minutes or so and last for sixty seconds. You are then usually completely effaced, or thinned out. Changing from between two and four centimeters to fully dilated during the active phase of labor takes an average of four and a half hours and is the most uncomfortable part of labor.

By the time you are dilated eight centimeters, you are likely to notice that your baby is descending in the birth canal. In this later part of the active phase, known as transition, there is often an urge to push, or bear down. This is a natural reflex and is experienced as an uncontrollable need to expel the baby by holding your breath and bearing down as though having a bowel movement. Most of the time doctors will discourage you from acting on this urge because the cervix is not yet completely out of the way. Unless your cervix is fully dilated, the pushing is likely to be ineffective.

Determining dilation is as much an art as a science. Patients often joke, "Why can't you tell how dilated I am with an X ray or an ultrasound?" The cervix is not visible on an X ray and can be seen only poorly by ultrasound. Even a pelvic exam by your obstetrician is not always completely accurate. Sometimes the cervix is far back in the vagina and difficult to feel. There is nothing more discouraging than to be told that you are now less dilated than you were last week or an hour ago. Your cervix did not actually shrink, but a subjective assessment of it might have changed.

The Second Stage (First Labor)

Your second stage of labor begins with complete dilation. Now you actively assist in the birthing process by bearing down, or pushing. While your contractions are still very strong and frequent during the second stage of labor, this stage is usually more bearable than before because you can now be an active participant. The baby is born on average within two hours of complete dilation. The actual pushing is done during contractions. You cannot meaningfully practice pushing before you need it. Your nurses and doctors will give you plenty of coaching when it is time to push. With the beginning of a contraction, you should take a deep breath and hold it for ten seconds while pushing with your abdominal muscles. After a ten-second rest, take another deep breath and bear down again. Most women are able to push three times during each contraction. While pushing, it is common to expel urine or feces, and for this reason, at the beginning of labor you may choose to get an enema to clear your rectum, though this is certainly not necessary.

The First and Second Stages in Subsequent Labors

There are some key differences in labor during your second and subsequent pregnancies. First, while the latent phase of labor can also last a long time, it is often much shorter after the first pregnancy, since you do not usually start this labor until dilation is relatively advanced. Second, the active phase of labor is also faster in second and subsequent pregnancies—an average of two and a half hours rather than four and a half hours. Finally, the second stage usually lasts less than one hour rather than up to two hours as with a first labor. All these factors combine to make a much faster and more bearable labor following the first pregnancy. Perhaps most important of all, second and subsequent labors are more unpredictable. It is not unusual for a woman pregnant with her second child to show up at the hospital dilated seven centimeters or, occasionally, completely dilated.

Although the second stage of labor is usually uncomfortable, most women manage to get through it with a minimum of medical assistance, particularly when they focus on pushing during their contractions. Recently I was making notes on a patient's chart when I heard peculiar shrieking from the adjoining delivery room where one of my patients was pushing in the final moments of her second pregnancy. She had been previously confined to her bed at home for eight weeks to help prevent preterm labor. Fortunately, she had made it to term. Since the noises coming from the delivery room were so strange, I decided to investigate. She was not shrieking with her contractions; she was actually giggling wildly between them!

"How can you be laughing during the end of labor?" I asked.

"Dr. Benson, I am so happy this pregnancy is over, I think this is just great." True to her moment of greatness, she delivered a healthy boy shortly thereafter. Some hours later, she still wore a smile of both relief and joy.

The Third Stage of Labor

This is simply the expulsion of the placenta after the birth. It usually takes only five minutes, rarely more than twenty. The only difference in the third stage between first and subsequent labors is that the cramping, or afterpains, after the placenta has delivered is more uncomfortable in the later pregnancies. After the placenta has been delivered, the nurse will often administer an injection of Pitocin to make the uterus contract. This helps to reduce vaginal bleeding after the delivery.

Chapter Three

THE BAG OF WATERS

The bag of waters, or amniotic membranes, fits the imagery of
medieval times as well as the space age. It can be viewed as a magic
cloak protecting the fetus from evil forces or as a controlled
environment for the fetus awaiting launch into the world in which
we live. In the language of modern medicine, the membranes
attach to the inner surface of the placenta and entirely surround
the baby, protecting it both from accidental bumps to the mother
and from bacteria, which may enter the womb from the vagina.
The water contained within the bag is called, logically enough,
amniotic fluid.

WHAT ARE RUPTURING MEMBRANES?

While "rupture" conjures up violent images, the membranes are
not part of the baby, and neither the baby nor you will feel any
discomfort from this event. Indeed, it can be such a subtle occurrence that both you and your doctor may be uncertain whether or
not the water bag is leaking. The size of the breach in the membranes is basically irrelevant, although a large leak is more obvious

than a small one. Once the membranes break, the potential exists for subsequent infection of the womb or even of the baby if your pregnancy continues for an extended period of time (days or weeks). There is no truth to the widespread belief that the baby has to be delivered within twenty-four hours of rupturing membranes.

Premature rupture of membranes (PROM) means that your water bag has broken before the onset of labor. It does not mean that the membranes have ruptured before term and that the baby will be premature. Spontaneous rupture of membranes (SROM) occurs when the bag of waters or membranes breaks naturally, without medical intervention. The procedure by which the doctor or nurse pokes a hole through intact membranes is known as artificial rupture of membranes (AROM).

There are three times during pregnancy when the water bag can break: (1) before term, (2) at term, before labor, and (3) during labor. Preterm premature rupture of membranes is unfortunate if it happens during the middle trimester, since this almost invariably results in a miscarriage, either from labor or the inevitable infection if labor does not occur. If the water bag breaks in the third trimester, before thirty-eight weeks, a premature infant usually results, again either from labor or from the need to induce labor due to infection. The consequences of prematurity vary greatly among individuals and are most dependent on the length of the gestation. In any case, less than 2 percent of women break their water bag before term.

Ten percent of women will have their water bag break at term before labor begins. Of these women, 80 percent to 90 percent will go into labor within the next twenty-four hours. For the few who do not, most obstetricians will recommend the use of medication to induce labor at some point to reduce the chance of a subsequent infection of the womb. Although the incidence of infection, or chorioamnionitis, is small after the water bag breaks, it slowly rises as days pass without delivery (see Chapter Eight on induction of labor).

While only 10 percent of mothers-to-be are destined to rupture membranes before labor, it seems that most worry it will happen to them. I remember one patient who had a recurring dream that she would experience a huge gush while shopping at the grocery store. In fact, her water bag broke spontaneously when she was in labor at five centimeters.

HOW CAN I TELL IF MY WATER BAG HAS BROKEN?

Amniotic fluid is a clear, watery liquid that will either gush or drip out of the vagina. Sometimes it may be difficult to distinguish it from urine. Indeed, you may realize that your water bag has broken during urination when fluid continues to pour out into the toilet after your bladder is empty. Once in a while you can distinguish urine from amniotic fluid because urine has an obvious ammonia smell. Alternatively, the only clue may be the constant dampness of your underwear. This can be very confusing since you will often have some dampness due to increased sweating unrelated to amniotic fluid close to term. The key is to notice a sudden change in vaginal moisture.

How can your doctor or nurse confirm that the water bag has broken? There are three methods commonly used. The first is a simple visual inspection of the vaginal opening, which often reveals whether the fluid is leaking from the vagina or the urethra. The second method involves testing the acidity of vaginal fluid with nitrazine paper. In 90 percent of women, the urine is acid enough to turn the paper green. In contrast, amniotic fluid is basic and will turn the paper a deep blue. The presence of blood or a vaginal infection can sometimes interfere with this test, but the test is usually helpful in distinguishing amniotic fluid from urine.

An alternative test involves touching a cotton swab to the fluid in the back of the vagina and smearing the swab on a slide. After the amniotic fluid dries, in a minute or two, it will appear as a fernlike pattern when viewed through a microscope under low power. If fluid does not leak out of the vagina on examination, a metal speculum might be inserted to permit a direct view of the cervix and access to the few drops of fluid from the back of the vagina. Even with the use of these three methods, the diagnosis may be uncertain. Usually the leak will recur over a few hours if your membranes are truly ruptured.

WHAT IS THE MUCUS PLUG AND BLOODY SHOW?

The mucus plug is often mistaken for amniotic fluid, but it is mucus secreted by your cervix that passes out of the vagina as the cervix softens in preparation for labor several days before contractions actually begin. The key to telling the difference between the mucus plug and rupture of the membranes is the fact that the mucus plug is thick and has the appearance of clear nasal mucus while amniotic fluid is watery. Sometimes the amniotic fluid may have little white speckles called vernix floating in it. Vernix comes from a protective layer of fat that is deposited on your baby's skin within the womb close to term.

Some people have heard that the mucus plug appears twelve or twenty-four hours before the onset of labor. While the mucus plug often is passed a few days before labor, sometimes it is seen weeks before delivery and many women do not ever see it.

Bloody show may or may not occur with the passage of the mucus plug. This is vaginal bleeding that occurs several days or hours before the onset of active labor. Usually it is associated with the passage of mucus as well, but it can be simply bright-red bleeding. Occasionally, bloody show results in rather brisk bleeding. However, any vaginal bleeding at term that requires the use of more than one or two pads per hour should be brought to your doctor's attention.

WILL MY DOCTOR BREAK MY WATER BAG IF IT DOES NOT BREAK ON ITS OWN?

When is the normal time for your water bag to break during labor? Anytime. In fact, on occasion, you may not break your water bag even as the baby delivers. It merely stretches and completely envelopes the baby. This is known as delivering in cul and is neither abnormal nor worrisome. If the membranes do rupture, you may experience a large gush during labor, or you may have only a small trickle. The gushing or trickling can continue throughout labor or there may be no further leakage after the initial flow. Keep in mind that there is no set pattern in the events associated with the water bag. The time at which the water bag breaks and the quantity of fluid that gushes forth are both highly variable. Just about any pattern is normal once labor has begun.

Why would your doctor or nurse want to break the water bag? There are several reasons. First, the more precise labor- and fetal-monitoring techniques require direct access to the womb or the fetus without intervening membranes. Second, since you are highly likely to go into labor within twenty-four hours after the water bag is broken, breaking the bag is one way to induce labor. Many physicians also think that breaking the water bag during an already established, slowly progressing labor may help speed the process. There is little scientific evidence for this belief, although practically everyone who delivers babies believes it. From my own experience, it certainly does seem to help speed labor in some. Finally, breaking the water bag is useful in establishing the presence or absence of meconium before delivery. Meconium is the substance that babies eliminate from their colons when they move their bowels within the womb. This will be discussed more fully later in this chapter.

How does your doctor break the water bag? This is a simple procedure. Your obstetrician identifies the cervix with one hand and with the other hand introduces into the vaginal canal a small plastic hook on a long handle. The hook is pressed against the membranes and then gently withdrawn, snagging the thin amniotic membrane and making a hole. Just like when the water bag breaks on its own, there may be a gush or just a small trickle of fluid. If the baby's head is firmly against the cervix no fluid may appear at first. The membranes can also be broken when a scalp electrode is applied to the baby's scalp directly through the amniotic membranes. The electrode will gently tear the membranes as they balloon with the pressure of contractions (see fetal monitoring in Chapter Four).

Is there a danger to the baby when the water bag is artificially broken? Basically, no. However, on those rare occasions when the baby's head is high in the pelvis and not firmly against the cervix, there is a small risk. Under these circumstances, a sudden rush of fluid out of the cervix could be accompanied by the umbilical cord falling in front of the baby's head and partially through the cervix. This is known as cord prolapse and is an obstetric emergency, since the blood flow through the umbilical cord is compromised when the baby's head puts pressure on it. Treatment for this complication is prompt cesarean section. This problem is rare and can even happen when the membranes break on their own. In my experience, I have not seen a cord prolapse even once whether I ruptured membranes or they broke spontaneously.

Of course, artificial rupture of membranes does commit you to delivery within the next few days to minimize the chance of a womb infection. However, this is rarely a major drawback since there is no reason to rupture membranes unless you are undergoing an induction of labor or are already in labor.

Some patients prefer that we do not rupture membranes unless it is absolutely necessary. It is necessary if we want to do internal monitoring, which is often the case when patients ask for epidurals. However, without an epidural, internal monitoring is often not necessary and we do not need to rupture membranes.

WHAT IS MECONIUM?

As mentioned above, meconium is the substance that passes from the colon if the baby has a bowel movement while still inside the womb. The material is dark green or black and consists of mucus, other secretions, and dead cells shed by the fetal intestines. Most babies do not empty their colon prior to delivery. If they do, the bowel movement can occur any time from days or weeks before labor to during labor itself.

How is the presence of meconium diagnosed? As you can imagine, if the water bag is intact, there is no easy way to tell if the baby has passed meconium. Once the membranes are broken, the diagnosis is relatively simple. Meconium will appear in the fluid leaking from the vagina as a dark green substance varying from thin and watery to thick and claylike. Thick meconium does not flow as easily as normal amniotic fluid and therefore may not emerge right away. On those rare occasions when the membranes are artificially broken and no fluid appears for hours, nurses and physicians may suspect the presence of thick meconium and take the appropriate measures described below.

If you feel fluid gushing or leaking from your vagina close to term, but it is dark green rather than clear, you should also suspect that your bag of waters has broken and notify your physician. Remember that the presence of meconium before labor is relatively unusual, while heavy vaginal secretions in pregnancy are common. Since some vaginal infections can result in an excessive discharge of opaque fluid, it may be confusing to know the source of the fluid. When in doubt, call your doctor.

What does the presence of meconium suggest about the baby's health, and what threat to the baby does meconium pose? The presence of meconium occasionally suggests a malnourished or sick fetus. In these cases, the meconium is usually thick, and there are often other factors that suggest a sick infant, such as poor fetal growth, or long-term maternal disease such as high blood pressure. The presence of meconium alone does not usually mean a jeopardized fetus, and most such babies demonstrate no abnormality during labor or at birth and beyond. The mere presence or absence of meconium is not particularly useful in predicting the health of your baby. Perhaps as many as 15 percent of normal-term fetuses pass meconium before delivery.

The second issue concerning meconium is the problem that it poses for the fetus at birth. As fetuses approach term, their attempts to swallow and breathe increase in frequency. Meconium that is passed within the bag of waters is rapidly distributed throughout the fluid. Inevitably, some of this material will enter the baby's mouth and upper airway passages. While this poses no threat before birth, there is a small risk to the baby at birth. Thick meconium can block the airways and can occasionally irritate the lungs and result in a sort of chemical pneumonia, but this type of problem is uncommon. Your obstetrician will try to eliminate any chance of difficulty by suctioning the airways well at birth. If meconium is present at birth, the nurses may also arrange for your newborn to have some physical therapy in which the infant's chest is gently tapped periodically to help loosen secretions. The presence of meconium is not a reason by itself to do a caesarean section, since your baby has to breathe no matter what the route of delivery.

Chapter Four

MONITORING LABOR

Labor in a hospital setting has always been monitored in the sense
that there was always a regular, formal evaluation of contraction
frequency and fetal heart rate. Prior to electronic monitoring, this
was done simply by placing a hand on the maternal abdomen
during a contraction and by listening to the fetal pulse with a
stethoscope. Now, with electronic monitoring, this is done with
machines. The advantage of electronic monitoring is that it is less
subjective and leaves a continuous written record of the contraction frequency and fetal pulse.

EXTERNAL CONTRACTION MONITORING

There are two effective methods for monitoring contractions.
The more commonly used method, the external tocodynamometer, is a device shaped like a hockey puck with a small bump
protruding from its middle. It is held onto your abdomen by an
elastic belt and is connected to the monitoring machine by a wire
approximately six-feet long. With each contraction, your abdomen tightens and the bump on the tocodynamometer is pressed

inward. This displacement is recorded on the monitoring device at the bedside on a scale from zero to one hundred. Simultaneously, a permanent record of your contractions over time is graphed by recording the changes sensed by the device. The contraction frequency and length can be instantly determined simply by looking at the graph paper as it moves through the machine. This method is more sensitive than the human hand in determining the relative strength and length of contractions but is still not as precise as we would like. The tocodynamometer is not very sensitive if a person is significantly overweight. It is most useful for making a permanent record of frequency and timing of contractions. These features are critical for meaningful interpretation of changes in the fetal pulse, which will be discussed later.

Is external contraction monitoring dangerous? Although this method has some limitations, it is not at all dangerous since it is an entirely passive form of monitoring and emits no energy such as ultrasound or X ray that could theoretically damage you or your baby. Its disadvantage is that the belt may be uncomfortable to wear for hours at a time. Also, the cord restricts walking while the monitor belt is being used. However, it can be easily moved and taken off from time to time, so these restrictions are not too important to most women.

INTERNAL CONTRACTION MONITORING

Occasionally a more precise method of contraction monitoring is required. Such precision is needed when there is suspicion that the uterine contractions are not frequent or strong enough or when the fetus has an abnormal pulse pattern. If it becomes necessary to have precise information on length and strength of contractions, your obstetrician will choose the internal monitoring method that utilizes a device known as an intrauterine pressure catheter, or IUPC.

An IUPC consists of a long, thin plastic tube with a small pressure sensor in its tip. It is attached to the monitor by a ten-foot cord. Your doctor does a pelvic exam with one hand to identify the cervix and then uses the other hand to slide the plastic tube inside the cervix. The tube is advanced for ten inches within the womb and then attached to a strain gauge. The entire process takes fifteen to thirty seconds and is no more uncomfortable than a pelvic exam during labor.

The IUPC uses a scale similar to that used on blood pressure cuffs, and records pressure in millimeters of mercury. These devices are much more accurate than any type of external monitoring because they rest directly within the uterus. When the womb contracts, the small computer chip at the tip of the catheter generates a signal that corresponds to the pressure inside the uterus. When the IUPC is functioning properly, the pressure within the uterus usually reads under 20 between contractions. Effective contractions will reach at least a pressure of 40 millimeters of mercury. In actual practice, some machines record a resting pressure of slightly over 20. Also, it is not uncommon for contraction strength to reach 80 at peak pressure.

What are the drawbacks associated with internal pressure monitoring? As with the external monitor, the IUPC limits movement, to some degree. It does not prevent you from urinating or moving your bowels. Also, the bag of waters must be broken and the cervix dilated to about two centimeters before the IUPC can be placed within the womb. It also has the theoretical disadvantage of increasing the likelihood of a womb infection following labor, although this is not usually a meaningful risk. In addition, when the IUPC is placed within the uterus, the small plastic tube can perforate the uterine wall. This occurs very infrequently because the catheter is soft and flexible. On the rare occasions when a perforation does occur, usually nothing untoward happens because the tube has a small diameter.

WHAT IS EXTERNAL PULSE MONITORING?

Just as with contraction monitoring, there are two common types of fetal-pulse monitoring methods: external and internal. External monitoring uses an ultrasound device held in place on your abdomen by an elastic belt. This device is approximately the size of a hockey puck and is connected to the monitor by a cord six- to ten-feet long. The belt is easily removed when you wish to walk. As your baby moves during labor, the monitor frequently needs to be readjusted to focus on the fetal heartbeat. Many machines have green, yellow, and red lights to indicate how well the monitor is picking up the fetal heartbeat. It is logical to assume that the red light is a warning signal indicating that the baby is in danger, but this is not the case. The red indicator simply means that either the baby or the monitoring device moved, preventing a good pickup of the heartbeat. All monitors have a speaker that allows them to broadcast the baby's pulse rate. In practice, this sounds like a fast thumping and can be quite tiresome after several hours. If you find the sound annoying, simply ask the nurse to turn down the volume.

The external monitor beams sound waves at the baby's heart and then detects the echo. As the heart walls pulse, the echo from the heart changes in frequency. The machine is able to determine the heartbeat rate on the basis of these changing echoes. In practice, the method works reasonably well, but it does have some flaws. For example, if the fetal heart rate is very slow, the machine tends to double it; if very fast, the machine will sometimes halve the pulse. Also, as will be seen, the machine is not as precise as an internal monitor. Finally, in the later stages of labor, as the fetus moves lower in the pelvis and the mother moves more with each contraction, the heart rate becomes difficult to monitor continuously. This is also the case when the mother sits up for an epidural anesthetic (discussed in Chapter Seven on pain relief). Even with these disadvantages, external monitoring is frequently all that is needed to assure fetal health during labor.

Fetal pulse is indicated by the monitor in two ways: through a flashing numerical display and by a continuous pen-tracing on a scaled strip of graph paper that moves through the machine at a constant rate. The heart rate tends to stay within the range of 120 to 160 beats per minute, although the pulse will be faster or slower at various points during the labor. The absolute number is not so important; it is the pattern of slowing down and speeding up of the pulse that indicates fetal health.

HOW DOES INTERNAL MONITORING WORK?

This type of monitoring is more accurate but requires that the amniotic membranes be broken. Thus it is not suitable for evaluating the fetal pulse before rupture of membranes. Internal monitoring determines the baby's pulse rate by measuring the electrical activity of the fetal heart through a wire attached to the baby's scalp. This method produces a continuous electrocardiogram similar to the monitoring of adults in coronary care or intensive care units.

Internal monitoring tends to provide a more precise heart rate than does external monitoring, because the electrical signal is easier to analyze than the changing echoes of the ultrasound device. Also, as the electrode is attached directly to your baby, the information continues despite movement by you or the baby during labor. The extra precision is required only in a minority of labors in which there is some question about the baby's health. Usually internal monitoring is used when you request an epidural anesthetic or during the later stages of labor when it is desirable to have a constant monitoring of the pulse.

An electrode is placed on the baby's scalp by your doctor or nurse during a pelvic exam. The head is identified with the examining hand while the other hand presses the plastic introducer containing the electrode against the scalp and then twists it half a turn. A tiny metal loop at the end of a wire then lodges in the baby's scalp. The introducer is then removed, leaving the wire trailing through your vagina. This wire is then attached to a small plate held in place on your upper thigh by an elastic belt. The thought of a wire passing through the vagina and being attached to the baby's head may be quite unappealing at first. In practice, internal monitoring often gives you more freedom to move and frees you of the occasionally uncomfortable external monitoring belt on the abdomen. It does not interfere with urination or bowel movements.

Several years ago it was common practice for parents attending Lamaze childbirth classes to reassure themselves that the wire did not hurt the baby by screwing the wire into their own hands. This practice soon lost its popularity when physicians warned that people could transmit a variety of infectious diseases to themselves. No doubt applying the electrode to the scalp is momentarily uncomfortable for the fetus. However, it is probably no worse than the blood draws newborns undergo for state-mandated screening tests.

WHO BENEFITS?

The human species has successfully produced generations of healthy adults without benefit of modern fetal surveillance during labor. But perhaps those few babies who do suffer injury during labor can be detected and helped. The pulse pattern shown by fetal monitoring is at least partially indicative of reduced oxygen supply or blood flow to the fetus. There are three basic types of problems that may be caused by limited oxygen to the fetus during labor: stillbirth, mental retardation, and cerebral palsy. Damage to other organs can also occur, but the fetal brain seems to be the organ most sensitive to reduced oxygen.

Let's examine each of these problems separately. Only one-third of stillbirths occur during labor; the majority occur before the onset of contractions. Monitoring might be able to prevent those stillbirths that occur during labor and delivery in only 2 to 3 per 1,000 deliveries. In addition, there is some evidence that monitoring can reduce the number of babies that die in the first week following birth, from 8 per 1,000 to 3 per 1,000. These reduced stillbirth and neonatal death rates may not be an unmixed blessing since very sick babies who might have died otherwise may survive, leading to a variety of permanent impairments.

What about prevention of mental retardation? Severe mental retardation occurs at a rate of 3.5 per 1,000 population; more mild mental impairments occur at roughly 25 per 1,000. Reduced oxygen supply during labor is thought to account for only a small fraction (perhaps 10 percent) of all forms of mental retardation. If monitoring is effective in screening for reduced blood flow and oxygen to the fetus, it would be expected to prevent retardation in only 3 babies per 1,000.

As with mental retardation, cerebral palsy seems to be only tenuously linked to deprivation of oxygen during labor. The National Institutes of Health (NIH) estimates that 25 percent to 50 percent of children with cerebral palsy developed the disorder during labor, although the most recent research suggests that problems during birth might account for less than 10 percent of all cerebral palsy cases. Conversely, only a small percentage of babies who have an impaired oxygen supply at birth develop cerebral palsy. Fortunately, it is less common than mental retardation, developing in only 5 infants per 1,000 births. The NIH suggests that monitoring might help some of the infants in this group: maybe an additional 1 or 2 per 1,000.

In the final analysis, if monitoring does screen for reduced fetal oxygenation during labor and obstetricians could use this information to intervene effectively, it could improve outcomes for roughly 13 per 1,000 newborns—about 1.3 percent. As a parent of an affected child whose outcome might have been different with continuous monitoring, this number is enormous. More than 98 percent of babies would probably derive no benefit from this surveillance. Furthermore, the mothers most likely to have an oxygen-deprived baby during labor can be identified as being high risk before they go into labor. These are mothers with high blood pressure, diabetes, preterm labor, and other problems due to their general health or the pregnancy itself. The benefit of continous electronic monitoring of healthy women with uncomplicated pregnancies has not been clearly demonstrated.

However, as is so often the case in medicine, if one child in several hundred could be saved from mental retardation or cerebral palsy, or kept alive as a result of fetal monitoring, it seems to matter little that most newborns derive no benefit from such monitoring. Almost all parents will do whatever they can to improve their child's well-being, and fetal monitoring is one way to help at least a few children. Most hospitals use electronic monitoring to some extent for all their patients in labor and delivery.

IS MONITORING DANGEROUS?

The risks are small and some are almost entirely theoretical, since monitoring has not been shown to cause frequent problems. With external monitoring, the fetus is exposed to hours of continuous ultrasound energy. At the frequency and level of energy used during labor, no significant biological effect from exposure has been demonstrated in the laboratory or in humans. While the potential harmful effects of X-ray radiation were not fully appreciated until decades after the introduction of the procedure, the use of ultrasound is not really similar. The energies involved in fetal monitoring are relatively small, and physicians have not discovered any harmful effects after several decades of such monitoring.

Internal monitoring has a different set of potentially adverse effects on the baby. This monitoring is entirely passive. Unlike ultrasound, the electrode emits no energy of its own; it simply detects the electrical energy given off from the baby's heart. However, local scalp infections have been reported in as many as 4 percent of the babies that have received internal monitoring. These scalp infections rarely require treatment other that a warm compress, and are usually limited to temporary redness and swelling where the electrode was applied. Infections requiring significant doses of antibiotics are rare.

A separate concern about internal monitoring has been the risk of infecting the mother. There is no good evidence to support the fear that placement of this wire within the mother's womb increases her chances of developing an infection. The probability of womb infection is much more closely related to the length of labor. In practice, the advantages of fetal monitoring seem to outweigh the risks.

WHAT DOES THE MONITOR TRACING MEAN?

Whether the monitoring method is internal or external, a pulse rate is plotted against time on graph paper that moves through the monitoring machine at a constant rate. This pulse rate has three important features that can sometimes indicate the adequacy of oxygen supplied to the fetal brain. The *baseline* is defined as the central beats-per-minute value around which the fetal heart rate varies. It is taken in ten-minute intervals. Normal values are a fetal pulse between 120 and 160 heartbeats per minute. However, pulses significantly faster or slower can be normal under many circumstances and are not generally a cause for alarm. The fetal heart rate in particular will rise if the laboring mother has a fever. Sometimes perfectly healthy babies have a pulse that is close to 200.

Variability is the frequent readjustment in the pulse rate of the healthy fetus. This results in a pronounced wiggle in the recorded tracing of the pulse. Constant readjustment is also reflected by the flashing numbers on the monitor, indicating that the pulse is changing speed. This is reassuring and suggests that the part of the brain responsible for control of the heart rate is getting adequate oxygen.

There are two types of *periodic changes*: accelerations and decelerations of the pulse for more than five seconds but less than one to two minutes. Accelerations occur spontaneously or with fetal movements and can sometimes coincide with contractions. These are almost always a sign of fetal well-being. Decelerations often result from temporary compression of the umbilical cord during labor and are to be expected. Slowing of the baby's heart beat can be of some concern, particularly if the slowing is less than 70 beats per minute for more than sixty seconds, but the worrisome decreases in the baby's heartbeat are rather rare.

Some general principles of monitoring are noteworthy. First, fetal monitoring is much more accurate in predicting a healthy baby than a sick one. Yet abnormal tracings are not infrequently associated with the birth of a vigorous infant. Also, an "abnormal" tracing can take hours to develop and often can be corrected through relatively simple intervention without resorting to immediate delivery. Second, many questionable aspects of the heart-rate tracings are resolved with time. Slowings in the fetal pulse are rarely worrisome by themselves and occur in the majority of labors at some point. In the vast majority of labors, the monitor tracing serves to reassure the doctor and the parents that the fetus is adapting well to labor.

WHAT HAPPENS IF MY BABY HAS A WORRISOME PULSE PATTERN?

When the monitor tracing suggests that the baby is not getting a sufficient supply of oxygen during labor, several steps short of immediate delivery are often effective. Simply having the mother change position, or giving additional fluid through an intravenous line, are often sufficient. You can also receive oxygen.

Rarely will an observed pattern require immediate action. For example, the prolonged slowing of the baby's pulse below 70 beats per minute for several minutes suggests that the umbilical cord is being squeezed. Under these circumstances, the cord is often wrapped around the baby's neck or some other part of the body or the cord may be momentarily compressed between the baby and the uterine wall. Whatever the cause, the pattern suggests that little blood is flowing through the umbilical cord to the baby. If this occurs, you will be asked to change your position, first to one side and then to the other in an effort to dislodge the cord. If the pulse does not pick up, your nurse or doctor will then do a vaginal exam to be sure that the umbilical cord is not coming out ahead of the baby. The examiner will gently push the baby up within the birth canal in an additional effort to free the cord. If all these maneuvers fail, an emergency caesarean section may need to be performed. Babies are not affected by cord compression that lasts only a few minutes, but might begin to suffocate if it persists for a much longer time. Fortunately, such severe and sudden cord compression is uncommon. It is estimated that one-fourth of all healthy babies born at term have the umbilical cord wrapped around their neck. I have personally delivered two vigorous infants with the cord wrapped around the neck *four* times.

The more usual pattern is for tracings to change slowly toward the abnormal. In these cases the issue is whether the baby will be born before its health is compromised. For example, if the tracing is markedly abnormal for at least half an hour and delivery is estimated to be hours away, your doctor may recommend a caesarean section. There will be instances, however, when labor can continue, particularly if the tracing is not too foreboding and delivery is anticipated in a short time.

Fetal monitoring may prove quite helpful even when it shows no problem at all. Anticipated difficulties may not occur, so planned interventions such as cearean section can sometimes be avoided.

WHAT IS A FETAL SCALP pH?

An additional test, the fetal scalp pH, is available for fetuses with questionable pulse patterns or with patterns that are difficult to interpret. By obtaining a drop of blood from the fetal scalp during labor, the pH, which is a measure of acidity, can be determined. If the fetus has not been receiving quite enough oxygen over a long period of time or if it has not been receiving any for a few minutes, acids will build up in the fetal bloodstream. While a small buildup of acid by itself is not harmful, it can indicate that the baby is not thriving in labor.

The pH of the blood taken from the artery of a healthy adult is 7.40. A normal fetal scalp pH is considered to be 7.25 and above. Values between 7.20 and 7.25 are borderline and generally should be taken again after a period of time. Values under 7.20 indicate that the baby should be delivered within thirty to sixty minutes to prevent possible harm from lack of oxygen, although obstetricians now suspect that a pH of less than 7.20 may still be normal in many cases.

Unfortunately, obtaining a scalp pH is not quite as easy as placing an electrode on the fetal head. In fact, the cervix must be dilated to at least three to four centimeters and, as with internal monitoring, the bag of waters has to be broken before the sample can be obtained. You will be asked to lie on your back or your side while your doctor places a hollow, cone-shaped piece of plastic into your vagina. This is not nearly as uncomfortable as it sounds.

Once the cone is firmly placed against the baby's scalp, the head is dried off with long cotton swabs. A clear gel is swabbed onto the fetal head, and the scalp is then nicked with a tiny razor on the end of a long, narrow handle. As a drop of blood accumulates, it is drawn up into a long hollow glass tube. Generally your obstetrician will try to get two such samples. With a little pressure on the scalp from a cotton swab, the bleeding stops and the procedure is over. The pH of the drop of blood is then analyzed.

Obtaining a scalp pH entails three to five minutes of moderate discomfort for the mother. Even so, the test can be an invaluable aid to your doctor in allowing him to decide that labor can continue. Since abnormal tracings predict a potentially compromised fetus with only limited reliability, the scalp pH is an additional test that allows the doctor to confirm that your baby is indeed stressed, or conversely, is not in jeopardy. While many babies are in good condition at birth even with a low pH, some may be in jeopardy and can benefit from prompt delivery.

What are the risks of sampling for pH? As with internal monitoring, a local scalp infection is a possibility, although this is almost never seen and when it is, it is rarely serious.

WILL MONITORING PREVENT ALL PROBLEMS?

Continuous fetal heart-rate monitoring during labor is a useful screening tool for the specific task of assuring that the proper amount of oxygen is being supplied to the baby. But a good tracing certainly does not assure a viable, healthy baby. It is possible for a profoundly impaired fetus to produce a normal tracing throughout labor. Fetal and contraction monitoring will help many babies but, sadly, not all.

Chapter Five

HASTENING LABOR

This chapter covers both labor induction and the use of forceps. Both serve to hasten labor, accomplishing a vaginal birth that might not otherwise take place. While forceps have been available for centuries, induction of labor with Pitocin as currently practiced is a relatively recent innovation.

WHY WOULD I NEED TO BE INDUCED?

The two most common reasons for inducing labor are premature rupture of membranes and postterm pregnancy. Roughly 10 percent of the pregnancies that go to term are complicated by premature rupture of membranes. As noted earlier in the discussion about ruptured membranes, this may be defined as rupture of amniotic membranes before the onset of labor. This is marked by a gush of fluid from the vagina or by the continuous leakage of a clear, watery fluid. Occasionally, if meconium has been passed, premature rupture of membranes may reveal itself by a dark green, relatively thick new vaginal discharge. Premature rupture should not be confused with the issue of delivering a premature baby. In this context, "premature" simply refers to the relation-ship of breaking the water bag prior to the onset of labor. When the membranes break at term, your baby will be delivered at term.

Eighty percent to 90 percent of women with premature rupture of membranes at term will go into spontaneous labor within twenty-four hours. The reason for this is not entirely understood. In fact, artificially rupturing membranes is one technique for inducing labor. This is also known as surgical induction of labor. It has not been shown to speed labor if the woman is already having relatively frequent contractions.

What if your membranes happen to rupture but you don't go into labor? Bacteria are not commonly found within the uterus or amniotic fluid during pregnancy. However, once the membranes have broken, the bacteria that normally inhabit the vagina have ready access to the uterine cavity. Given enough time and the proper conditions, they can overwhelm the womb's defenses and cause a significant, potentially dangerous, infection. An infection with the baby still inside the uterus is known as chorioamnionitis. A persistent postpartum infection of the womb that remains after the birth of the baby is called endometritis.

Chorioamnionitis at term fortunately does not often result in serious harm to either you or your baby, as long as the baby is delivered relatively promptly. The infection can become serious if the delivery does not take place for several days. In most cases, it is readily curable in you and your baby with antibiotics. The diag-nosis of chorioamnionitis can be relatively difficult to make. No lab test, symptom, or physical finding will completely confirm the condition. Physicians suspect an infection if you have a fever, a rise in pulse, a tender uterus, or if the baby's pulse rises in the presence of prolonged rupture of membranes.

If you do not go into labor following premature rupture of membranes, doctors have two options. They can either wait longer for labor or induce labor with oxytocin. If your doctor waits, the risk of chorioamnionitis increases with time. If you are induced and the cervix is not somewhat dilated or thinned out, the induc-tion may not work, necessitating a caesarean section. The probability of a so-called failed induction rises significantly with a cervix that is not substantially thinned out or dilated.

There are no good studies that clearly identify the best single course of action that your doctor should take. Specifically, the risk of infection with time following rupture of membranes is not well established, although it seems to increase. There is some evidence that there is not much harm in waiting even days, as long as the mother does not develop a fever. As a result, many physicians wait twelve to twenty-four hours for labor to begin if the cervix is not ripe (somewhat dilated and effaced). For women who are already significantly dilated, there is not much benefit to waiting, since induction under these circumstances rarely fails.

The second commonly encountered reason for induction of labor is postterm pregnancies. These are not pregnancies that merely go past the due date—they must go at least two weeks past the date. Here, too, the issue of failed induction has a prominent role to play. A postterm woman with an unfavorable cervix (poorly dilated and effaced) undergoing induction has a significant risk of requiring a caesarean section for failed induction. As the days pass awaiting cervical effacement, the risk of stillbirth rises.

At forty-two weeks and beyond, physicians obtain tests of fetal well-being to be sure that waiting for the cervix to ripen is safe for the baby. The nonstress test uses external monitoring to establish a healthy fetal pulse pattern over the course of twenty to thirty minutes. An alternative test, the oxytocin challenge test (OCT), uses low doses of oxytocin to cause a brief episode of contractions during a ten-minute period. This test is reassuring if there is no significant slowing of the baby's heartbeat during this time. With the reassurance of one or both of these tests, you and your doctor may be content to await softening and dilatation of the cervix to make induction of labor more likely to succeed.

HOW WILL MY DOCTOR INDUCE LABOR?

Curiously enough, one of the greatest advances in obstetrics in the last century, the identification and production of the hormone oxytocin, has been the subject of considerable controversy in the past two decades. The manufactured version of oxytocin, Pitocin, is the drug that brings on labor. How does induced labor differ from "natural" labor? What are its dangers?

Oxytocin is a small protein hormone manufactured in the part of the brain called the hypothalamus, and is secreted by the pituitary gland. A pharmaceutical company has been able to synthesize oxytocin in very pure and large amounts. The company called its product Pitocin. Pitocin is practically identical to the naturally secreted hormone. Prior to the development of Pitocin, animal tissues with less pure forms of oxytocin were ground into tablets. Whenever a physician wanted to induce labor, he gave the woman a tablet, which she held in her mouth against her cheek. Enough of the drug was usually absorbed so that labor began. With current methods, small amounts of pure oxytocin are given intravenously at a constant rate.

With regard to the infusion itself, a somewhat intimidating pump is used to carefully regulate the flow of oxytocin into the veins. These computer-guided pumps can operate on either wall current or on batteries. The pumps are equipped with an alarm that signals when the infusion runs out or when there is an obstruction to the free flow of fluid into the vein. This occurs whenever the intravenous line is kinked. Since pumps usually blink a light or a number and occasionally make noises, they do not improve the atmosphere within the labor room. They greatly improve the safety of the oxytocin infusion, however, and for that reason should be welcomed.

The amount of oxytocin in the blood does not appear to rise significantly during labor until delivery is imminent. The level rises remarkably after birth. This is thought to help cause the uterus to contract strongly to reduce the amount of postpartum bleeding. Also, the release of oxytocin with suckling during breast-feeding is thought to be responsible for milk letdown. As many pregnant women have observed, nipple stimulation before labor will actually result in contractions, due to oxytocin release.

There are three ways in which an induced labor differs from natural labor. First, natural labor can often take hours or days to develop into hard labor. Characteristically, the contractions can come and go every fifteen to thirty minutes until a strong, regular pattern is attained. With oxytocin, the interval from a woman's first perception of cramps to hard labor is often only several hours.

Second, induced labor tends to be somewhat shorter than spontaneous labor, probably due to the way the oxytocin is administered. The intravenous infusion rate is increased every fifteen minutes until contractions occur approximately every three minutes. While the contractions in many naturally occurring labors come every three minutes, in many women they can occur slightly less frequently. It has been suggested that the arbitrary three-minute goal may be modestly more frequent than the rate at which contractions occur in spontaneous labor. If the contractions do occur with somewhat less rest time in between, at least the labor ends that much sooner. While the contractions may seem to be somewhat stronger than natural contractions, more recent data suggests that there is little difference in the peak pressure or length of contraction itself. The most supportable conclusion, therefore, is that oxytocin does make contractions occur more frequently, but they are probably not stronger than with regular labor.

The third way that induced labor differs from natural labor is that many physicians are much more liberal about prescribing pain medication with the infusion of oxytocin than without it. Some give narcotics or an epidural with the first request for pain relief during an induction regardless of cervical change or absolute dilatation. With spontaneous labor, many obstetricians wait to give narcotics until cervical change has occurred, and delay the epidural until the woman is dilated four to five centimeters, hoping to avoid slowing labor with their interventions. Once you are already receiving oxytocin, however, if the contractions space out, we merely increase the infusion rate. As a result, many doctors see no disadvantage in giving pharmacologic pain relief as soon as it is requested since any change in the frequency of contractions is easily remedied.

In addition to using oxytocin to induce labor, doctors may also use it to augment labor in a woman whose cervix has already begun to dilate and efface. Your obstetrician may use Pitocin commonly to augment labor if your cervical dilation is abnormally slow. One common reason for slow dilation is epidural anesthesia. For reasons poorly understood, contractions often diminish in strength and frequency after the anesthetic is administered. At a nearby hospital whose statistics I am aware of, 40 percent of women who ultimately delivered received oxytocin at some point in their labor. As epidural anesthesia becomes more popular, Pitocin augmentation will no doubt become more common.

The chief danger of oxytocin is that it can cause excessively frequent contractions and thus reduce the blood flow to your baby. Contractions every two minutes, or contractions for more than 50 percent of the time, are commonly known as tachysystole. Tachysystole can also occur in spontaneous labors. Whether it occurs in induced or natural labor, it rarely compromises the baby. If it does occur with induced labor, the oxytocin supply can be turned down and the tachysystole will rapidly disappear. With the continuous fetal monitoring performed during the oxytocin infusion, the fetus is watched closely for any evidence of compromise. Finally, the widespread use of electronic infusion pumps to control the amount of medicine delivered to the maternal blood stream adds an extra margin of safety.

When has an induction failed? Most obstetricians do not think an induction has failed until oxytocin has been infusing for a number of hours after the rupture of membranes without cervical dilatation, although sometimes it may be impossible to rupture the membrane. For those women who are postterm with unfavorable cervices, a two-day induction may be considered. On the first day, the oxytocin is given for twelve hours or so and then stopped overnight if the cervix is not significantly dilated by the end of the day. On this first day, particularly with first pregnancies, many women barely feel the contractions. On the morning of the second day, the doctor then breaks the bags of waters and begins the oxytocin again. Even for women with unfavorable cervices at the outset, this method is usually effective in producing a good labor pattern.

WHAT ARE FORCEPS AND HOW ARE THEY USED?

As with induction of labor, forceps can be used to hasten delivery or even accomplish a delivery that might not otherwise occur. Hundreds of years after the development of the forceps, their use has become controversial. Proponents of forceps argue that their judicious use can help cut down on the rising caesarean section rate. Others point out that the increased safety of caesarean section obviates the need for forceps.

The first metal instruments used for extracting babies in a vaginal delivery were described in the medical literature during the early twelfth century. From the teeth on their inner surfaces, it seems pretty clear that these instruments were meant to deliver only stillbirths. An English physician, Hugh Chamberlen, is generally credited with being most responsible for their design and subsequent widespread use by the early part of the seventeenth century. This was almost three hundred years before caesarean birth provided a viable alternative to vaginal delivery. Before this time, failure of the fetus to deliver in a reasonable time period invariably meant stillbirth. If the dead fetus did not deliver subsequently, the mother frequently died as well. In the era before caesarean birth was reasonably safe, forceps saved many mothers and babies.

In the 1990's, forceps deliveries have to be judged by a different criterion of success. With survival of the mother virtually taken for granted, and fetal survival assumed in most uncomplicated pregnancies, the good health of the liveborn is now of paramount importance. It is most significant that a prominent obstetric text notes that "Except for two specialized forceps . . . very little that is both new and useful in obstetrics has been added to the development of the instrument in over 200 years" (*Williams Obstetrics*, sixteenth edition, 1980).

An outlet forceps delivery consists of applying the forceps to the fetal head when the scalp is visible through the labia between contractions. Low forceps refers to placement when the fetus is low in the birth canal but the scalp is not quite visible. Midforceps delivery entails assisting a fetus that is engaged in the pelvis but not too far down the birth canal. High forceps delivery, no longer done for safety reasons, was done before caesarean sections were a reasonable alternative, and involved applying forceps before the fetal head was engaged or "locked" into the pelvis. Low forceps deliveries, in which the fetal scalp is not quite visible, are actually rather easy. Midforceps deliveries are often more difficult, for instance when the fetus has to be rotated more than ninety degrees in order to deliver.

A forceps delivery is relatively straightforward. Placing the forceps on the baby's head within the birth canal is rather uncomfortable for you, so your obstetrician will probably suggest one of the anesthetic techniques discussed in later chapters, such as an epidural or a caudal anesthetic. Occasionally, a pudendal block, which is the injection of local anesthetic near nerves next to the vagina, given by the obstetrician proves adequate. Once the anesthetic has been administered, your doctor carefully places the forceps on the baby's head. With the next contraction he gently tugs as you do your best to push. Together, you guide the baby through the last one or two inches of the birth canal. As one obstetrician I know is fond of saying, "There should be no 'force' in forceps."

Babies born with forceps assistance generally have mild bruising over the cheeks that last for a few days. Lacerations or tears of your vagina are not infrequent with forceps, although most are easily repaired. Infrequently, forceps can damage the bladder or rectum, necessitating surgical repair.

Are forceps deliveries safe? Low forceps and easy midforceps deliveries do not increase the risk to the fetus. Infant outcomes following more difficult midforceps deliveries yield controversial results, both short and long term. For this reason, many obstetricians prefer to have women push longer during the second stage rather than apply forceps prematurely.

Over the past several decades, an alternative to forceps, the vacuum extractor, has been developed to assist vaginal birth. This procedure involves placing a plastic suction cup on the fetal head, turning on a pump to create a mild vacuum, and then applying gentle traction to ease the fetus down the birth canal. With the current plastic suction cups and the hand pumps in wide usage, fetal risk is minimal, as the suction cup will slip off if too much traction is used. Other than temporary bruising on the scalp where the vacuum is applied, the vacuum does not leave marks on the newborn. Vacuum extractions tend to result in fewer tears of the birth canal than do forceps deliveries.

Chapter Six

"PREPARED" CHILDBIRTH

This chapter is the first of three dealing with pain relief during labor and delivery. Your preparation prior to having your baby may be an important contributor to reducing, though not eliminating, the pain of childbirth. Thus, prepared childbirth is logically the first topic to be reviewed when dealing with the general subject of pain in labor and delivery. Since prepared childbirth may mean different things to different people, and is often viewed as synonymous with "natural" childbirth, some definitions are in order.

WHAT IS IT?

Prepared childbirth means preparation for childbirth, whether reading this book, learning and doing special exercises, or attending Lamaze classes. I believe, as do most obstetricians, that any type of sound preparation for childbirth is beneficial, and the more, the better. If hospital procedures are known in advance, and if you are better able to understand the reasons for your doctor's actions during the labor and delivery process, the entire hospital experience will be less stressful or anxiety-provoking.

Among the various methods of preparation for childbirth, the one most widely taught is Lamaze. It is easy to learn, effective, and not prone to cause women to feel guilty if they require pain medication. Other childbirth-preparation methods such as Bradley and Gamper are similar to Lamaze in that they stress education and provide activities that tend to distract the laboring woman during contractions. Due to its popularity, a large part of this chapter is devoted specifically to the Lamaze method.

Taken literally, natural childbirth suggests to me the image of a woman giving birth in a field—that is, without medical personnel nearby. When some of my patients request natural childbirth, they might mean that they hope to avoid asking for pain medication. For a few this means that I should not even ask them if they want pain relief during labor. Others use the term simply to express their hope that they deliver vaginally or without the need for an episiotomy (described in Chapter Eight). It is probably best not to use the term natural childbirth at all, since it has so many different meanings. Most women who give birth do not require any significant intervention by their obstetrician. The vast majority of mothers give birth in the hospital in order to have access to pharmacologic pain relief and other forms of medical assistance, should any be needed.

Occasionally obstetricians see patients who are literally over-prepared. One patient presented us with a three-page typed list of instructions for her labor. We did our best to abide by the list, which included the instructions not to ask her if she wanted pain medication however uncomfortable she might be. Unfortunately, her fetus hadn't read the list, and he had grown to a good size during pregnancy and simply could not fit through the birth canal. Ultimately the woman received an epidural for labor discomfort (at her request) and was delivered by cesarean section. Preparation always helps, but keep in mind that the experience itself may be quite unpredictable. Be ready to throw away your script and ad lib your way through labor.

HOW BAD WILL MY PAIN BE?

What about the pain of labor and delivery? The Bible is extremely clear about this issue, as God admonishes Eve in the Garden of Eden: "I will greatly multiply thy pain and thy travail; in pain shall thou shalt bring forth children . . ." (Gen. 3:16). Obstetric texts are equally dire in their predictions, since many state that the pain of labor for the expectant woman will, in many cases, "be the most painful event that she has ever experienced."

Numerous studies have demonstrated that women in labor suffer significant pain, regardless of culture, race, or ethnicity. One recent study from McGill University in Montreal provides particular insight into the pain of labor. Psychologists there developed a sixty-two-point pain-scoring system. With this system, 60 percent of women in their first labor described their pain as severe or unbearable. As expected, the figure fell to 35 percent of women with subsequent labors. Further, researchers found that childbirth preparation reduced perceived pain somewhat, but not nearly to the extent of that provided by an epidural anesthesia.

This conclusion deserves emphasis. Some women who are about to have their first baby announce at the outset of labor that the hospital staff should not ask them if they want any type of pain relief because they will not need it. Then when they subsequently plead for narcotics or an epidural, they feel guilty. They tend to believe that somehow they have failed as mothers even before their babies are born. This makes me sad. Laboring women should not grade themselves as mothers on the basis of whether or not they require pain relief.

Several important truths regarding the pain of labor are worth noting. Most important is that a first labor is usually longer and more painful than subsequent labors. Second, among women experiencing first labor, the degree of discomfort varies widely. Though the "average" description of a first labor and delivery is one of severe discomfort, some women have relatively fast and minimally uncomfortable births. Also, while a woman's attitude and preparation may have a profound effect on her perception of the experience, her pain is neither imagined nor simply an experience that occurs because society has come to expect it.

The fact that women may experience markedly different levels of pain during childbirth has at least one interesting consequence. It means that the experiences of a neighbor or relative may provide little insight into what you are likely to experience. Often women who have relatively little pain look askance at those who cry out or complain of the severe pain. It is inappropriate to judge the conduct of others in this situation, especially since the level of pain from woman to woman can vary substantially.

I recently heard a humorous interchange between two of my patients. I was making an entry on a medical chart nearby when one mother whom I had just delivered bumped into one of my other patients in early labor. The mother-to-be at the end of her first pregnancy was anxiously plying her new acquaintance with questions, grasping for any clue that would predict what lay ahead. I couldn't help but smile when the mother who had just delivered urged the laboring mother to ask for Pitocin. "Why, I had my baby in four hours and I barely felt a thing!" she said. While this was true, she forgot to mention that she was induced for being overdue and that she began labor at four centimeters dilated. She also didn't point out that her previous two labors were fast ones also. For labor, someone else's experience doesn't always provide a good idea about what to expect.

Why is labor so uncomfortable for most women? No one knows for sure. While medical theories abound, the best way to understand this pain is to compare it with other painful conditions. Doctors universally recognize that one of the most severe pains in the human condition is that from an "obstructed hollow viscus." This is a muscular tube that is contracting against insurmountable resistance. Examples include the passage of a kidney stone, gall bladder attacks, and the intense pain of a bowel obstruction. Labor consists of a hollow muscular tube, the uterus, contracting in an effort to expel the baby against the significant resistance of tissue and bone. Labor by its very nature is painful, whatever the biochemistry involved.

There are two features of childbirth that fortunately help to make it much more bearable. First, labor is a physiologic process that is an inextricable part of female gender identification. That is, from the time of their own birth, most women grow up fully expecting to go through labor as a normal part of womanhood. While most of us do not expect to develop kidney stones, a painful condition whose presence is not consistent with good health, labor is a normal, healthy, long-anticipated event. Second, an even more important consideration is that labor ends with the birth of a baby—a momentous and joyous experience. So while labor may be painful, it is virtually the only physiologic process involving severe pain that is associated with both good health and a good outcome.

HOW DOES LAMAZE WORK?

How, or perhaps why, does the Lamaze method help women through labor? Most important, Lamaze training presents a thorough discussion of what can be expected during childbirth, so that both parents can feel in control of events rather than controlled by them. Also, Lamaze uses a type of self-hypnosis that serves to focus the laboring woman's attention away from the discomfort of contractions.

Hypnosis is an intensely focused state of concentration. People vary in their ability to be hypnotized, that is, to concentrate on one thing to the exclusion of everything else. All of us have some capacity to have our attention focused on particular thoughts and sensations and focused away from others. Women with Lamaze training are able to breathe through their contractions in a special way, guided by their husband or partner. They and their spouses are taught special massages to help with contractions. They also learn to concentrate on a focal point, some interesting picture or object brought from home. These activities all give the woman something to do during contractions other than lying in bed with her attention focused solely on the pain of labor.

Many women with Lamaze preparation request pain medication with their first labor. Lamaze still has value for these people, since they are much better able to tolerate labor in the early and late stages, when medication may not be appropriate. Lamaze preparation should not be seen as a substitute for pain medication but rather as an adjunct to it. Obstetricians and labor and delivery nurses can walk into a laboring patient's room during a contraction and usually know immediately whether or not the patient has had childbirth-preparation classes. Patients with preparation tolerate labor better, with or without drugs.

Of course, sometimes Lamaze preparation is all that is needed. Recently, a patient committed to minimal intervention announced during a prenatal visit that she would not require pain medication before labor. While normally we regard such a statement as an almost certain jinx, she was true to her word. She concentrated on a picture of her husband holding their new puppy and was able to do Lamaze breathing throughout her labor. She turned down our offers of something to "take the edge off" and delivered a healthy girl after a labor of average duration. Prepared childbirth does allow some people to make it all the way through without help, but there is no shame if it does not provide total relief.

WHAT DOES LAMAZE INVOLVE?

During active labor the contractions last an average of one minute. Usually there are two minutes of rest between contractions. This time can be used to prepare for the next contraction. With this in mind, there are basically four Lamaze skills to be mastered.

First, the focal point is a specific object that you look at while you do your breathing during contractions. During your last month of pregnancy, pick out some colorful, familiar object at home and bring it with you when you go to the hospital. During contractions, concentrate on looking directly at this object, studying it while you do your Lamaze breathing. Photos of pets, children, husbands have all served well in this capacity. For some reason, I have yet to see someone use a photograph of their doctor as a focal point.

Second, there are several types of massages that are helpful during labor. Most can be performed by yourself, although your

husband can also help. Effleurage is a fingertip massage that begins
with both hands placed together just above the pubic bone. With
your fingertips, apply gentle pressure as your hands move upward
and outward toward the hips. This can be done ten to twenty times
during the minute-long contraction and does not need to match
the rate of breathing.

Another type of massage taught in Lamaze class is stroking.
This massage is often of great help. Gently stroke your thighs and
arms with your hands while relaxing the part of your body that
you are massaging. Sometimes you will prefer back and shoulder
massages during strong contractions so that you are distracted
from your abdomen. This can be particularly helpful during back
labor, in which the most intense discomfort is along the lower
spine.

Third, Lamaze instructors also emphasize relaxation. They encourage you to relax your lower pelvic muscles and provide less
resistance as your baby passes through the uterus. Much of the
resistance to the baby's passage is provided by your bony pelvis and
pelvic and lower abdominal musculature, which is out of your
voluntary control. Nevertheless, relaxation can be beneficial, particularly during the pushing or second stage of labor and as the
baby crowns. It is also helpful since it tends to prevent you from
tensing your entire body during a contraction and thus tiring
sooner.

In the same manner that you actively tense a muscle, you can
actively relax it. A clenched fist can be slowly and deliberately
unclenched. This is different than simply allowing the fist to go
limp. Active relaxation can be practiced and refined in brief
sessions twice daily. How can you do relaxing exercises? Any drill
that helps reduce tension in all or part of your body should suffice.
While you are on your back, you can raise one leg while relaxing
the opposite one. This also can be done with your arms. In the
same position, you can alternately contract and then relax toes,
feet, ankles, calves, and then thighs, first with one leg and then
with both. Practicing these types of relaxation exercises in advance will help you reduce your physical tension during labor. You
will tire less as a result.

The fourth Lamaze technique is breathing. There are five special types of breathing that are used for labor and delivery. Most contractions begin gently and then rapidly gain strength. Occasionally, contractions begin with great intensity. The breathing methods described below should be adapted to the strength and pattern of each individual contraction.

The cleansing breath is a very deep breath taken in through your nose and blown out through your mouth. Inflate your lungs as completely as possible with the intake. Begin and end each contraction with a cleansing breath. It helps to prevent hyperventilation and aids in relaxation.

Early labor breathing is deliberate, deep breathing though not as deep as the cleansing breath. Inhale and exhale air through your mouth. As this breathing is practiced, you can see your chest rise and fall.

Stronger labor breathing is used as the contractions become more uncomfortable. Begin each contraction with a cleansing breath. As the contraction builds in intensity, take several deep early labor breaths. At the peak of the contraction, which usually lasts from twenty to thirty seconds, breathe through your mouth rapidly and shallowly while you expand your chest moderately. When the peak of your contraction passes, end your deep breathing with a cleansing breath.

Transition breathing is desirable at the stage of labor known as transition, when the contractions that dilate the cervix from seven centimeters to the full ten centimeters tend to be particularly intense. Sometimes you will get an involuntary urge to push or bear down as the baby's head descends in your birth canal. Since it is often better to delay active pushing until the cervix is completely retracted out of the way of the baby, this part of labor is particularly trying. Transition breathing is the same as for stronger labor breathing except that with every fifth shallow breath at the peak of the contraction, make a special effort to blow out, or exhale forcefully. This helps to give rhythm to your breathing and serves to guard against hyperventilation. As the height of the contraction passes, switch to deep, shallow breathing, and end your contraction with a cleansing breath.

At complete dilation, you can speed delivery and shorten the period of your discomfort by actively pushing the baby through the birth canal. With the onset of a contraction, take a cleansing breath. Hold the next deep breath for ten seconds and then fully exhale. As you hold your breath, tighten your abdominal muscles, simultaneously bearing down as though you were straining at a bowel movement. With another deep breath, repeat this cycle. You are usually able to get in three good pushes with each contraction. The end of the contraction should be marked with a deep cleansing breath. A key to effective pushing is that it must be entirely silent. No air should escape through your vocal cords while the breath is held. Instead, guide the air downward to help push the baby through your birth canal.

Within one minute of birth, your doctor will ask for smaller pushes so that the vaginal tissues have a chance to stretch out of the way of the baby. This lighter pushing at the very end is not difficult to master since birth is only moments away.

WHAT IF I JUST CANNOT DO LAMAZE BREATHING?

Some women feel inadequate during labor if they do not perform according to certain preconceived notions. There are several reasons why a woman may depart from the Lamaze approach. First, people vary greatly in their ability to be hypnotized. As a result some women will be quite ineffectual in applying the techniques through no fault of their own. Second, some laboring women will experience more intense pain than others. If this pain causes you to scream, it will cause a breakdown in Lamaze breathing. Physicians and nurses assign no badge of merit to the nonscreamer who may just be having an easier labor.

Aside from screaming, you may momentarily lose concentration and breathe too quickly. You can tell this is happening if you begin to feel dizzy and your hands and feet tingle at the height of a contraction. While it is not dangerous for either you or your baby, most people prefer not to be dizzy. To stop the dizziness simply slow your breathing. If a contraction is overpowering and non-Lamaze breathing occurs despite diligent preparation, you should feel no embarrassment or concern.

IF I TAKE LAMAZE CLASS CAN I STILL ASK FOR PAIN MEDICATION?

Lamaze techniques do not prohibit the use of pain medication. With or without childbirth preparation some women will want other types of pain relief and some will not. No pain medication will be ordered by your obstetrician or nurse unless they believe it to be safe *and* you ask for it. The medical staff will not judge your dedication to motherhood on the basis of whether you are able to tough it out. This is an individual decision that can only be decided after the onset of labor. It is a choice that is dependent on your personal circumstances and should carry with it no guilt or remorse.

Chapter Seven

PAIN RELIEF DURING LABOR

Recent medical advances have made the administration of pain relief during labor much safer for women and their babies. The two basic types of relief are injectable medications and epidural anesthesia. Pain-control techniques do carry small risks, but are generally so safe that it is quite reasonable for you to request them during labor whenever you feel the need.

WHICH DRUGS CAN I ASK FOR DURING LABOR?

All of the medications commonly used for relieving pain during labor are narcotics. They are closely related to morphine and can cause addiction when misused. As prescribed for laboring patients, however, addiction is never a problem simply because we do not use the medications for days at a time. While the names of the drugs are different and include Demerol, Dilaudid, Fentanyl, morphine, and Stadol, their effects and side effects are largely the same. They vary in potency and speed of onset, but these are not important differences. The potency of a drug simply refers to the amount required to achieve a desired effect. For example, Dilaudid is more potent than morphine, so doctors prescribe less of this drug to achieve the same effect. To you as a patient, it hardly matters whether your obstetrician prescribes 1.5 milligrams of Dilaudid or 10 milligrams of morphine, since the amount of pain relief you experience should be identical.

With regard to the speed with which the drug takes effect, narcotics that are injected into the vein relieve pain more rapidly than medications injected into muscle (in the buttocks or arms). However, the drug also dissipates more rapidly when injected intravenously. The various narcotics have slightly differing speeds of onset, but your doctor adjusts for this by modifying the route of administration and frequency of dosing. Sometimes the narcotic is administered in a split dose. Part is given through the intravenous line directly into the circulatory system while the rest is injected under the skin or into the muscle. The intravenous dose is active within minutes and has a short duration while the injected drug takes effect more slowly but typically lasts longer. After several doses of a narcotic during labor, each subsequent dose is slightly less effective. Finally, all of the narcotics have similar potential side effects. If you experience nausea with one drug, you will not necessarily develop the problem with another. It is difficult to predict in advance how you will respond. The majority of patients notice significant benefit without being troubled much by side effects. If one drug bothers you, we simply switch to another.

Narcotics provide relief by changing the way the brain perceives pain. To this end, they are used routinely in the hospital for surgical patients and others with significant pain. In labor, they also modify rather than eliminate the perception of pain during contractions. While you are aware of the fact that you are having a contraction, the discomfort is much more bearable.

WHAT ARE THE SIDE EFFECTS AND DANGERS OF PAIN MEDICATION?

A small percentage of the population develops nausea in response to any one of these drugs, particularly when they are used for postoperative pain relief. Since nausea during labor is quite common anyway, it is sometimes difficult to tell whether you are nauseated from the drug or from labor. Another side effect is sedation or drowsiness. This effect is usually mild, and you are unlikely to fall asleep during labor. Some people are also allergic to the narcotics and can develop rashes or other reactions, although this is infrequent. The side effects and dangers of the drugs appear minimal with the amounts commonly used for pain relief.

Can the drugs harm my baby? Several considerations are raised by this question. First, it is not possible for a drug administered during labor to cause birth defects, since it is given no earlier than a half day before birth. Nevertheless, these drugs cross the placenta to enter the fetal circulation, resulting in fetal sedation. They do not impair your baby's blood or oxygen supply while in the womb, and their effect is largely a scientific curiosity. This may not be true if the drug is given within an hour prior to the baby's birth. Sedation at time of birth may result in a sleepy baby who has decreased respiration.

Although sedation of the baby sounds worrisome, it is much less threatening than it appears. Poor respiration is relatively common in the early minutes of life even among babies who have had no sedation. Medical personnel who work in labor and delivery are very familiar with helping babies breathe by giving them puffs of oxygen through a mask placed gently over their faces. Also, an injection of a drug called Narcan will within seconds completely reverse the sedative effects of any narcotic the fetus has absorbed. For these reasons, sedation poses very little risk to your baby.

There is an interesting beneficial effect of narcotics and other types of anesthesia. Preliminary evidence indicates that drugs that reduce the pain of labor may increase the blood flow to the uterus and, in turn, the supply of oxygen to the baby. The significant discomfort of labor releases adrenaline into the bloodstream, which tends to cause a constriction of blood vessels, including those that supply the uterus. Pain-relief medications may diminish this adrenaline release and help improve blood flow to your uterus.

The narcotics, in particular, may have an additional beneficial effect. Some researchers suggest that the narcotics may help to slow fetal metabolism when they pass through the placenta to the baby. If this is the case, the fetuses of mothers that receive narcotics may consume oxygen less rapidly. As a result, they may actually have increased protection against the reduction of oxygen supply during labor. Though the evidence for these beneficial effects is preliminary and tentative, these findings suggest that pain medication during labor may not just be safe but may actually be of benefit to the fetus in addition to making the mother more comfortable.

When will pain medication be given to me during labor? The answer is whenever you ask for it, as long as there is no health reason not to give it. As a rule, we avoid prescribing narcotics if you are in very early labor—before you are several centimeters dilated—because narcotics may slow the contractions in this stage. Also, if the drug is given too soon, the subsequent doses are less effective when you need pain relief more urgently. As noted above, we try to avoid prescribing the drug just prior to delivery. If prescribed closer to birth, we will specify a reduced dose.

Many patients tell us during their prenatal visits that they do not want us to give them any pain medication unless they "need" it. Pain medication is never needed. It is never given to make labor safer, only to make the mother more comfortable. Obstetricians and nurses will not give you pain medication unless you ask for it.

Occasionally, husbands and wives get into disputes over whether the wife should take pain medication. The matter is fairly easy to resolve because as long as you are conscious, you are the one who either accepts or declines pain medication, whatever well-meaning family members suggest.

WHAT IS AN EPIDURAL ANESTHETIC?

Also known as the Cadillac of anesthesia for laboring women, the continuous lumbar epidural involves administration of an anesthetic agent through a small plastic tube that rests along the spinal cord. This eliminates the sensation of contractions and often results in such a high degree of comfort that you can sleep during the height of labor. To give you an epidural, the anesthesiologist first scrubs your back with a special soap and numbs an area over your backbone by injecting a local anesthetic through a small needle just under your skin. He then inserts a larger needle in between the lumbar (lower back) vertebrae until it rests just short of the sac containing the nerves that run through the backbone, or spinal cord. The region outside this sac, or dura, is called the epidural space, meaning *next to* the dura.

Once the needle is in position, a small plastic tube is threaded through it to rest within the backbone along the spinal cord. When the tube is in position, the needle is removed and the tube is taped firmly in place on your back. After a small dose of medicine is given to test your reaction to it, a larger dose is administered through the sealed end of the tube. It takes an average of ten to twenty minutes for you to experience significant pain relief.

This local anesthetic bathes the sac containing the main nerves of the lower body, resulting in numbness usually from the lower ribs down. Since the sensory nerves are easier to numb than the motor nerves, you are often able to move your legs at least partially, although you cannot feel them very well. With the tube securely taped to your back, you can get additional anesthetic without having to have another needle puncture. There are two ways to keep you comfortable indefinitely with the epidural catheter (or plastic tube). A fresh dose of medication (also known as a bolus of anesthetic) can be given whenever you begin to feel contractions again, or an electronic pump can be attached to the tube so that a constant flow of medication is given (continuous infusion method).

THE EPIDURAL SOUNDS GOOD! WHEN CAN I GET IT?

What is the common practice for administering epidurals during labor? Many obstetricians prefer to wait until the cervix is four or five centimeters dilated before having the anesthesiologist administer the anesthetic to those patients who request it. This wait is required because epidurals can occasionally slow contractions in early labor. Each dose will usually last for up to two hours. One or two additional doses are often given at the patient's request to provide pain relief if she is not yet fully dilated. Many doctors want the anesthetic to wear off by the time of the second stage of labor because they believe that the anesthetic may interfere with the push reflex. When your baby is very close to being delivered, you can be redosed with a special, short-acting anesthetic so that you do not experience the discomfort of delivery. If you are receiving a continuous infusion of epidural anesthetic, occasionally you will be able to feel enough of your contractions so that you can push effectively. If this is the case, your obstetrician may not stop the medication.

With an epidural you are fully conscious throughout labor and delivery. This anesthetic does not provide any sedative effects. If you are on your second labor or beyond, you will frequently have such a fast labor that an epidural cannot be given in time to provide appropriate pain relief. But then again, this is true only for short labors that do not require the same relief as your longer first labor. If you require a cesarean section, and already have the epidural catheter in place, you simply can get a slightly larger dose of anesthetic. This can save you a second anesthetic procedure just for the surgery.

IS AN EPIDURAL DANGEROUS?

Dangerous compared to what? The risk of death in one year from smoking is 1 in 200, from using an automobile about 1 in 6,000.

As I tell my patients, an epidural is an elective procedure that is done to make life more comfortable. By almost any standard, an epidural is safe. The risk of death or serious injury is much less than from driving a car for a year and even less than simply being pregnant. Yet there are potentially dangerous complications from an epidural. There are basically three types of risks to the mother: prolonged labor, the wet tap, and the bloody tap.

There is a great deal of controversy in the medical literature over whether epidural anesthesia lengthens labor. I suspect that it probably does. Everyone who works in the obstetric ward is aware that contractions occasionally seem to space out in the hour or so after an epidural is given. While the mechanism of this is poorly understood, it seems to occur with some regularity. Most obstetricians do not consider this a big problem because it is easily remedied with medication (Pitocin) to bring the contractions closer together. Also, mothers who are numb and cannot feel their contractions seem to take longer to push the baby out. This problem does not seem too troubling. Either we let the epidural anesthetic wear off or we simply wait longer for the baby to be born. Most mothers and babies are no worse for the wait. Occasionally, if someone has been pushing for hours, we might assist the birth with the vacuum or forceps, but this is not usually necessary.

If the epidural needle is inserted too far, through the dura membrane into the sac of nerves, a wet tap results. This is usually simple to diagnose because spinal fluid leaks out of the epidural needle or because the physician can feel the needle going through a membrane. Since the sac now has a hole in it, there is a small chance of a spinal headache developing. This headache can be mild or severe and can last for several days. When a wet tap is recognized, the needle is withdrawn and the procedure ended without the administration of medication. Some anesthesiologists may reattempt the procedure in a different location along the woman's spine, if she is so inclined.

There is effective treatment for a spinal headache, which works more than 95 percent of the time. It is known as the epidural blood patch. Several ounces of blood drawn from the patient's arm are injected into the epidural space in the vicinity of the anesthetic site. Relief is often immediate but can take up to a day. Though the spinal headache is rare, it is rather easily treatable. The great majority of epidurals provide successful pain relief with no spinal headache.

An unrecognized wet tap occurs when the anesthesiologist puts the epidural needle into the spinal sac but does not know it. If the anesthesiologist does not recognize that he has entered the dural membrane, he will proceed to inject the dose appropriate for an epidural, which is much more medicine than for a spinal. An overdose of anesthetic results and the patient can be numb from the neck down. A temporary paralysis usually results, which may prevent the laboring mother from breathing. If this occurs, the anesthesiologist will either manually assist the patient with her breathing or place her on a ventilator until the drug wears off. Although mother and baby usually suffer no ill effects from this experience, it is certainly an unwished-for event.

If the epidural needle enters a vein, thereby causing a bloody tap, blood will leak out of the needle and the anesthesiologist will withdraw or reposition it. On very rare occasions, the needle will enter a blood vessel or the plastic tube will shift slightly, penetrating a blood vessel. If the anesthetic enters the blood stream, the patient can have a seizure.

Several methods are used to recognize wet and bloody taps and thereby avoid any complications. First, when the needle is thought to be in the proper location, a syringe is attached and the plunger withdrawn. This will suck any blood or fluid into the syringe, where it will be easily visible. Second, a small test dose of medicine is given before the full dose. If this small amount is inadvertently injected directly into the circulation, the patient will experience tingling and a strange taste in the mouth. If this occurs, no additional drug will be given. With each additional dose of medicine, the syringe will be attached to the plastic tube. Again the plunger will be withdrawn to be sure that no fluid or blood comes out of the tube. These measures are effective in preventing problems.

HOW WILL IT AFFECT MY BABY?

What risk does the epidural pose for your baby? None, directly. The dose of medication for an epidural simply does not enter your circulation in sufficient concentration to affect the fetus. This is obvious, although few people realize it. Mothers with epidurals are fully conscious and have no clouding of their mind—the effect of the anesthetic agent is limited by its location near the nerves in the spine. It does not spread all over the body. However, the epidural is prone to lower blood pressure because it numbs the nerves from the pelvic blood vessels as well as from the sensory nerves. As a result, the blood vessels tend to dilate and cause a decrease in blood pressure. This can lead to lessened blood supply to the uterus and the fetus. Even if this occurs, the majority of fetuses are unaffected by the temporary decrease in blood flow. Decreases in maternal blood pressure have been linked to behavior changes such as weak sucking for up to forty-eight hours after birth. The fetuses that are most threatened by a reduction in blood pressure are already ill or malnourished. For this reason epidurals are not the pain relief of choice for women with compromised fetuses.

To avoid the problem of lowered blood pressure when you receive an epidural, increased amounts of fluid are added to your circulation through the intravenous line. This is effective in preventing a significant drop in pressure. If the blood pressure were to fall, despite the addition of fluid, medicine can be administered that will correct the drop in less than one minute.

WHAT IF I DO NOT WANT ANY DRUGS? IS THERE ANYTHING ELSE I CAN DO?

There are two other pain relief methods in which patients occasionally show some interest. The first is known as TENS, or transcutaneous electrical nerve stimulation. This technique involves attaching to various points along your spine skin electrodes that are connected to a battery-powered electric pulse generator.

When a contraction begins, you activate a switch that produces a low-intensity charge. The mechanism may be similar to the relief you experience when you rub a painful area of skin. In theory, the nerves that are activated with the rubbing stimulus send impulses to your brain that serve to block out the pain signals. Some studies have found that this method does not work any better than placebos, although other investigations have shown that TENS provides excellent relief for backache experienced in the first stage of labor. It is not useful for reducing the discomfort of delivery. The few patients of ours who have used this technique reported significant benefit, although they did not have particularly long or difficult labors.

An alternative pain-relief technique is acupuncture. In Chinese hospitals 20 percent to 30 percent of surgery is performed with this method alone or with some sedation. Thin needles are placed in an average of eight places on the body, providing anesthetic effects in twenty minutes. A key problem with using this method is that Chinese women have not traditionally used acupuncture for pain relief during labor. As a result, there is relatively little knowledge of the best locations for needle placement. Also, this method severely restricts the laboring woman's movement since the needles must remain undisturbed for best effect.

OKAY, DOCTOR. WHAT DO YOU RECOMMEND FOR ME?

For every risk of a medical intervention, there is a risk associated with nonintervention as well. Ideally, your obstetrician will act only when the risk of failing to act is greater. Pain medication for labor is one exception to this idea. There are basically no risks to *not* receiving pain relief and both narcotics and epidural anesthetics have risks. The key idea here is that the dangers of these methods are small enough so that it is reasonable to get pain relief, if only to improve the quality of life for a few hours. We take greater risks on a daily basis even if we do not recognize it. As noted earlier, driving a car for a year is much more dangerous than receiving either narcotics or an epidural anesthetic during labor. In a study of children four years after their birth, developmental status was unaffected by the method of pain relief given to the mother during labor. This study included children whose mothers did not receive any type of medication before their birth.

What do I recommend? Have an open mind. No matter how smart or experienced you or your doctor are, neither of you can predict what your labor will be like. The women who seem to have the most satisfactory experiences during labor play it by ear, so to speak. They do not announce beforehand that they will or will not need pain medication. They simply see how things go during labor. No one receives narcotics or an epidural without specifically requesting it, and when someone asks for pain relief, the nurses and doctors are usually eager to please. It is a rare exception in which health considerations prevent us from giving either narcotics or epidural anesthesia.

Chapter Eight

THE MOMENT OF BIRTH

Hours of labor are eclipsed by the excitement and tension at the moment your baby is born. This momentous event in your life occurs quickly; the baby takes only sixty seconds to pass through the vaginal opening. In the vast majority of cases, the events that transpire during and right after delivery are quite routine as you and your baby join together outside the womb for the first time.

WHAT TYPES OF ANESTHESIA ARE AVAILABLE FOR MY DELIVERY?

There are a variety of options for pain relief during the actual delivery. The most common by far is an injection of anesthetic directly into the skin where an episiotomy will be performed, if needed. There are different types of regional anesthetics, such as the lumbar epidural, which typically numb an entire region of your body. These anesthetics provide good pain relief while allowing you to witness the birth with a clear mind. The general anesthetic that puts you to sleep is reserved for rare emergencies.

If you had been given a lumbar epidural earlier, it can be redosed just before the delivery when you are done with most of the pushing. This effectively eliminates discomfort as your baby emerges from the birth canal. A delivery epidural may be associated with some increased chance of requiring outlet forceps (an easy forceps delivery), but this is a minimal disadvantage.

A single-dose caudal epidural anesthetic can be injected in the same manner as the lumbar epidural. Lumbar and caudal refer to specific parts of the lower spine, with the caudal region lying below the lumbar area. With the caudal epidural, the injection is made lower in your back so that the distribution of pain relief is more directed to your lower abdomen and pelvis than with the lumbar epidural. This method is effective in providing pain relief for delivery. Its risks are similar to the lumbar epidural and are small. Since this offers only one-time pain relief, it has largely been replaced by the lumbar epidural with catheter placement for repeated or continuous dosing.

The pudendal block consists of an anesthetic injection by your obstetrician into the region of the pudendal nerves. These nerves run along the walls of your pelvis on either side and supply sensation to the vagina and nearby regions. This anesthetic can significantly reduce the pain of childbirth but will not affect your sensation of contractions. Typically it is given ten to twenty minutes before the anticipated time of birth. It generally requires ten minutes to take full effect and lasts for forty-five minutes, which affords pain relief during the repair of the episiotomy or any lacerations that may occur.

To give you the pudendal, your doctor will examine you with one hand while holding a syringe and needle in the other. Once the appropriate bony landmark on one side is identified, the doctor makes two injections into the vaginal wall close to the path of the nerve. This procedure has to be repeated for the other side. Unfortunately, the pudendal does not always work on both sides, since the anatomical location of the nerves can vary. The injections themselves are uncomfortable for only a moment.

There are few risks with the pudendal. The principal concern is that the anesthetic will be inadvertently injected into the major blood vessels that usually run close to the nerves. If enough drug reaches the bloodstream in this manner, serious medical problems could occur. But just as with the administration of the lumbar epidural, the risk of this happening is slight. In both instances, great care is exercised in using these drugs. With the small amounts of anesthetics given in each injection, complications from pudendal anesthesia are very rare.

The local is the most commonly used type of anesthetic technique and is simply the injection of the agent directly into your skin to numb a limited, specific area. It is usually administered just before an episiotomy is made or when tears in the birth canal need to be repaired. The anesthetic will not significantly relieve the overall discomfort of either the contractions or the delivery. As with any anesthetic, injection into the blood vessels is always a risk, but there are no major blood vessels in the area where the local anesthetic is commonly injected. Also, the dose given is small.

WILL I NEED AN ENEMA?

Some aesthetic concerns are relevant at this point. Fortunately, you are no longer exposed to the complete prep—a total shaving of all your pubic hair. The only preparation that is commonly done now is simply to wash your external genital area with an iodine solution before the birth. During pushing and particularly during the birth itself, it is very common for you to lose urine and move your bowels. Your nurses and doctors often applaud this mess as proof of effective pushing. The mandatory enema in early labor fell by the wayside once it was viewed as being convenient for the doctor only, not for the patient. Some women prefer an enema in advance, because whatever stool is in the rectum during labor will be forced out.

WHAT ABOUT STIRRUPS?

Another practice that is now mostly condemned is placing women in stirrups at birth. The comfort and position of the stirrups vary widely with different delivery tables. They all require the woman to deliver with her legs widely separated and flexed at the knees. Some patients tolerate this position well, but others do not. Other possible positions include squatting, standing, and lying on the side. Relatively few women seem inclined to squat or stand during the birth itself but some find lying on their side to be of benefit. Usually stirrups are most helpful when it comes to repairing the episiotomy or any lacerations after delivery. Stirrups on delivery beds manufactured in the past decade resemble modified footrests.

WHAT ABOUT DAD?

When I was born, my father was no closer that one hundred yards away and on a different floor of the hospital. Today, we actively encourage fathers to remain with the delivering mother both to provide support and to participate in the birth directly. Most fathers are happy to do so. Many are naturally nervous at first about what they will see. Understandably, they hate to see their mate in discomfort. Occasionally, fathers or even women themselves suggest that dad wait outside. This is a good idea for those who faint or feel exceptionally nervous. For fathers who remain at the birth, the degree of involvement varies and is a matter of personal preference. I have let fathers deliver their own babies, though few wish to do so. For my own children, I did not even want to cut the cord, since I was too busy holding my wife's hand and taking pictures.

Once the baby is delivered, many hospitals arrange matters so that the parents are not separated from their newborn unless the mother wishes to rest. The baby is weighed and receives his or her first bath in a separate recovery room to which the mother is also moved. Occasionally this is all accomplished in a combination labor and delivery room.

WHAT ABOUT THE LEBOYER BIRTH METHOD?

The French physician Dr. Leboyer and his ideas about natural birth have added additional controversy to the mechanics of birth within the modern obstetric suite. Dr. Leboyer advocates, among other things, dim lights and prompt, warm-water baths for newborns. Some people think that the way the baby is delivered and his environment at the moment he is born will somehow have a long-term effect on his development and personality. There is no doubt that the birthing process for the baby is not one of life's more comfortable moments. But to suggest that the noise and lights outside of the birth canal can in some way adversely affect the baby for life is difficult to support with facts.

WHAT HAPPENS TO ME AT DELIVERY?

Typically your baby is initially positioned in the womb so that he faces your side. As he moves down the birth canal he rotates so that he is looking toward your backbone. With descent, the head is flexed forward so that the baby's chin touches his chest. This enables the smallest diameter of the head to pass through the pelvis. As the head is pushed toward the vaginal opening, the scalp begins to bulge through your labia, an event called crowning. This process can take some time with the birth of a first baby. With a second baby, only a few minutes may elapse between crowning and birth. The crowning process allows the fetus to stretch the vaginal opening enough so that he can pass through it.

As your baby is born, the head passes through the vaginal opening usually facing your rectum. When the head emerges from the birth canal, it rotates either to the right or the left, back to the same position it was in before the delivery. Your obstetrician then uses a bulb suction to suck out the baby's mouth and nose, after which the soon-to-be-born infant often takes his first breath—even before his shoulders have passed out of your body. With one more push, the baby is born, as first the upper shoulder slides under your pubic bone, and then the lower shoulder passes out in front of the rectum.

WHAT IS A POSTERIOR BABY?

In 5 percent to 10 percent of cases, the baby will face toward the ceiling and not toward the floor. This is known as sunny-side up, or posterior. The position of the baby might impinge on the quality of labor but poses no health risks. Sunny-side up babies are popularly associated with uncomfortable back labor. If you experience this type of labor, you will feel your contractions primarily as back pain. I am not convinced that back labor is inherently more uncomfortable than contractions felt in the front of the abdomen or that back labor is primarily or even commonly associated with so-called posterior babies. As mentioned in previous chapters, it is very difficult to compare levels of discomfort among women.

As labor progresses, many posterior babies rotate as they move down the birth canal so that they are facing downward as they emerge. This rotation process, however, can add several hours to labor, allowing time for the baby to slowly corkscrew through the pelvis, and may lengthen the time necessary for you to push the baby out.

WILL MY BABY'S BELLY BUTTON POINT IN OR OUT?

Many people wonder what the obstetrician does to make the umbilicus point in or out. Nothing the obstetrician does affects the way the umbilicus points. This is completely dependent on the local tissue strength of the baby. We do not tie the umbilical cord nor do we have any control over the cosmetic appearance of the umbilicus in later life. Perhaps years ago it was common practice to actually tie it off with suture material, but currently we simply put a plastic clamp on it and cut off the remainder. The five minutes immediately following the birth of the baby have in the past generated much controversy. Most of the assertions about appropriate actions to be taken during this period have little practical importance anymore when considered in the light of modern medicine, but there is debate in some quarters as to when to cut the umbilical cord. If your doctor does not intervene, the cord will normally stop pulsating and seal within three to five minutes. We often clamp and cut the cord shortly after birth so that your baby can be promptly dried and swaddled.

There is also some debate about whether to hold your baby above or below the level of your abdomen for the first minute of life. This controversy stems from the fact that blood will either drain out of or into the baby depending on how high he is held. Since babies usually have an abundance of blood at birth, it almost never matters if a little blood drains away into the placenta when he is held up for his parents to see immediately after birth. Some people are concerned about holding the baby too low. They are fearful that if extra blood is allowed to transfuse into the baby from the placenta, the baby may actually have so much blood that it may not be able to circulate smoothly. These concerns are rarely of practical importance. For most doctors and nurses, the parents' wishes regarding their first contact with their newborn are of paramount importance. The obscure and largely outdated arguments concerning where to hold the baby and when to cut the cord should not interfere with a joyous experience.

WILL I NEED AN EPISIOTOMY?

There is some disagreement among obstetricians about whether an episiotomy should be performed. The episiotomy, made just prior to delivery, is a surgical incision in the skin between the vagina and the rectum to create a larger opening in the birth canal for the baby to pass through. There is little scientific evidence to indicate that the episiotomy helps either you or the baby at the time of birth or later in life. Of course, there is also little evidence to the contrary. Most obstetricians will do an episiotomy when the skin seems likely to tear. As a result, the majority of patients receive an episiotomy for the birth of their first child. For the second baby, the birth canal stretches more easily and episiotomies can often be avoided.

The majority of women will tear the skin between the vagina and the rectum with the delivery of the first baby. Before the advent of appropriate suture materials, most of these tears eventually healed by themselves. Although it may make sense to repair naturally occurring tears, the efficacy of cutting the skin to avoid having it tear is more controversial and less obvious. Some proponents of the episiotomy claim that it speeds delivery and reduces blood loss. Others suggest that a clean surgical incision rather than a jagged tear leads to stronger tissues in later life with a reduction in prolapse (falling out) of the uterus and bladder in post-menopausal women. Again, there is no scientific evidence for this claim, and I personally do not believe it. The few studies that have examined these issues found no decrease in average blood loss or delivery time. To be fair, no one really knows because an appropriate scientific study of these issues is inherently difficult.

There are reasons to perform an episiotomy that do make sense, lack of evidence notwithstanding. On many occasions a well-planned incision in advance seems to prevent a larger, naturally occurring tear. Many physicians also point out that a straight surgical incision is easier to repair than a jagged one. If you are likely to tear at delivery there is another reason to do an episiotomy, one that is seldom discussed. If you do not receive a delivery epidural, the area in which the episiotomy is to be made is numbed in advance with a shot of local anesthetic injected directly into the skin. This not only numbs the skin for the incision but also provides local anesthesia for the suturing of the wound after delivery. With the proper placement of anesthetic agent, both the incision itself and its repair are minimally uncomfortable for you. It is more difficult for your doctor (and more uncomfortable for you) to numb the edges of a jagged tear after the fact. At the least, the surgical incision probably helps to limit the size of the tear.

Virtually all obstetricians use dissolving sutures to sew up birth-canal tears or episiotomies. Two types are commonly used: specially treated catgut, which dissolves in seven to fourteen days, and the newer, synthetic sutures, which dissolve in fourteen to twenty-eight days. Some doctors prefer using the longer-lasting suture because they feel there is less inflammation (and pain) with this material. Others prefer the catgut sutures because there is less chance that they will be around in four weeks, when the new parents are given the go-ahead to resume lovemaking.

There are two basic types of episiotomies: the median or midline episiotomy and the mediolateral episiotomy. The midline episiotomy is the smaller of the two and hurts less while healing. This entails a small cut at the back of the vagina down the middle. The second and larger incision begins at the middle of the back of your vagina but is slanted off to the side. There is some debate about which type is better. However, the length of incision and pain of healing are not the only considerations here. It is not always easy to tell just how much room your baby will need at birth. As a result, a small episiotomy sometimes tears or "extends" further than the original cut. This is only occasionally a problem. If a small midline episiotomy is extended by a tear, it could tear right into the rectum. A mediolateral episiotomy, on the other hand, is less prone to such a tear since it is angled away from the rectum.

What happens when the rectum is torn at childbirth? Fortunately, this is not as bad as it sounds. Instead of the usual ten or fifteen minutes required to repair most tears and episiotomies, this type of laceration takes thirty to forty-five minutes to sew. Despite what you might imagine, this injury to the birth canal is usually not much more uncomfortable during healing than repairs of episiotomies or lacerations.

If you experience either an episiotomy or a tear, there are several types of pain relief available. First, an ice pack placed over the wound helps reduce the discomfort and swelling for the first day. Subsequently, warm tub baths several times a day seem to help healing and allow you to keep the area clean. Pain medication, such as Tylenol with codeine, is also offered as well as a local anesthetic spray. Nursing mothers can safely use this medication.

The discomfort usually subsides rather rapidly so that after a week your vaginal tissues are not too sore. Most physicians recommend that you wait four weeks or so before the resumption of intercourse. By this time you are usually well healed. Of course, if intercourse is very painful, abstain until your doctor inspects the episiotomy during the postpartum checkup.

Some people who deliver babies take pride in the fact that they can often avoid the need for an episiotomy or repair of a laceration. They simply hold the head of the baby back as the skin around the vaginal opening stretches. By delaying the delivery for several contractions (five to fifteen minutes), they give the skin a chance to stretch and are often able to avoid tears. Some of them take this action despite the fact that the last ten minutes of labor are extremely uncomfortable. It is not clear to me that prolonging the worst part of labor is worth it to avoid an episiotomy. In any case, if you prefer this, it is certainly no trouble for your obstetrician to allow the tissues to stretch rather than to cut them, although sometimes they will tear anyway.

WHAT IS THE AFTERBIRTH?

The delivery of the placenta is known as the third stage of labor. This stage usually takes twenty minutes or so, and comes right after the birth of the baby. The natural delivery of the placenta causes little discomfort since it is one-sixth the size of the baby and does not contain any bones. It is important that the entire placenta be expelled from your womb since any pieces left behind can lead to infection or additional blood loss.

When I was in my first year of private practice, I usually encouraged parents to look at the placenta. After the first two dozen couples turned away from it, I stopped pointing it out. It can be very interesting as often the amniotic membranes are still attached and you can get a good idea of your baby's previous abode. The rare, curious father will even photograph it.

Sometimes the placenta takes longer to deliver. It may be slow to separate or it may be trapped in a shrunken birth canal. In these instances, your doctor can reach in and remove it. Though seldom necessary, this manual removal can be quite uncomfortable, but it takes only thirty seconds. Some obstetricians "explore" your uterus by inserting a hand to be assured that part of the placenta has not been left behind. In most cases, though, the placenta comes out intact and the uterus does not need to be checked internally.

If the placenta is removed with difficulty and bleeding continues, a gentle scraping of the inside of the womb (a dilatation and curettage, or D and C) may be necessary to remove the remainder. You might be given general anesthesia for this procedure if you do not already have an epidural in place, as this relaxes the uterus and makes it easier to recover the placenta. The procedure takes only a few minutes and does not prolong the recovery from childbirth.

While a retained placenta is one cause of excessive bleeding after the birth, another cause is known as uterine atony. This simply means that the uterus fails to contract strongly enough after the baby and afterbirth have been delivered. An easy way to treat it is simply to rub the lower part of the abdomen. This is relatively uncomfortable but quite effective in making the uterus contract and thereby stopping the bleeding. Several different medications are also available to aid uterine contraction after birth. Postpartum contractions are not as strong as those during labor.

The average amount of blood lost from a totally normal birth is roughly a pint, or the amount that is given when donating one unit of blood. If you do not have enough iron in your diet, you will become anemic over the course of the pregnancy because your baby is the first to receive whatever iron is available in your body. Obviously, if you start out being anemic and then lose blood at delivery, your anemia will worsen. It is important for you to be conscientious in taking prenatal vitamins, which contain iron, and to eat properly. Any anemia present during this period can be detected by routine prenatal lab work.

Chapter Nine

WHY OBSTETRICIANS PERFORM CAESAREAN SECTIONS

WHY ARE MORE CAESAREAN SECTIONS BEING DONE?

The rate at which caesarean sections have been performed in recent years has risen sharply. In 1970, the caesarean section rate in this country was approximately 5.5 percent of total deliveries. By 1978, the rate had risen to approximately 15 percent. Currently the rate is about 24 percent nationwide but even higher at some hospitals. Obstetricians will sometimes justify this high caesarean section rate by pointing to the dramatic fall in the perinatal death rate. On the other hand, one Irish hospital reported a similar fall in the newborn death rate while holding the caesarean section rate constant at 4 percent to 5 percent. This may well mean that we are doing too many caesarean sections in this country.

There are several reasons for the fast-rising caesarean section rates during recent years. Of the most important causes of an increased rate, studies indicate that the largest single reason is dystocia, which is failure to progress in labor. This accounts for roughly one-third of the increase. One-fourth of the increase in caesarean section rate is repeat caesarean section. About 10 percent to 25 percent of the rise can be attributed to an increase in the delivery of breech (feet or buttocks first) babies by cae-sarean birth. Finally, the increasing rate of diagnosis of fetal intolerance to labor over the past decade accounts for 10 percent to 15 percent of the rise in the surgical delivery rate. An exam-ination of several of the indications for caesarean section will help you understand the pressures pushing physicians toward caesarean section.

WHAT HAPPENS IF THE BABY IS JUST NOT COMING?

There are three possibilities to consider if you do not seem to be making steady progress in labor. First, perhaps your contractions are not strong enough or frequent enough. Second, maybe you and your doctor simply need to wait longer. The third possibility is that your baby simply will not fit through the birth canal.

The chief treatment for poor progress in labor is waiting. Not everyone's labor proceeds like a graph in a textbook. Progress can be notoriously slow in early labor, before you are four centimeters or so dilated. However, if your doctor thinks that you should be further along than you are, the next thing he will consider is your contraction quality. To evaluate this better, your obstetrician may suggest placement of an IUPC (intrauterine pressure catheter), which can more accurately assess the contractions than external monitoring. If the contraction pattern seems unsatisfactory, you may benefit from medication such as Pitocin to make the contrac-tions more frequent.

If an expectant mother is four centimeters dilated or more, is having good contractions every three minutes, but is making no progress for at least two hours, her obstetrician will start thinking about the possibility that the baby simply will not fit. "Baby too

big to fit" is known in medical jargon as cephalopelvic disproportion (CPD). With CPD, it is hard to know if your baby is too big or
your pelvis is too small. In any event, the baby simply does not
deliver. Caesarean sections for cephalopelvic disproportion fortunately are rarely emergencies. Whenever the diagnosis is in
doubt, your obstetrician can apply the first treatment described
above, waiting some more. Occasionally, further progress will be
made after a temporary pause.

It is easy to see that the number-one reason for doing cae-
sareans today, cephalopelvic disproportion, will characteristically
result in operative delivery after a long labor. Patients often
ask afterwards why they had to go through all that just to
get a caesarean. Without seeing how things go during labor,
obstetricians simply have no way to know if vaginal delivery is
possible or not. Most women are able to deliver even a large baby
vaginally.

Your doctor will be the first to admit that fetal-weight assessment by examination or even by ultrasound is little better than a
guess. Recently, I asked one of my patients who was eleven days
past her due date to get an ultrasound for amniotic-fluid volume
and estimated fetal weight. The ultrasound suggested that the
fetus weighed 9 pounds 12 ounces. My exam gave a similar result as
I thought the weight was 9½ pounds. A few days later the woman
went into labor and delivered without any difficulty. The baby
weighed 7 pounds 15 ounces. Even if the weight had been correct,
I had no reason to believe that things would have turned out any
differently.

Not only is the diagnosis of cephalopelvic disproportion responsible for one-third of all caesarean sections, it has increased at the
fastest rate in the past twenty years. It appears that one reason this
diagnosis has become more common is a corresponding drop in the
use of midforceps. That is, rather than deliver a baby vaginally
with the use of midforceps, obstetricians are increasingly resorting
to caesarean section. A study at my hospital showed that a forceps
delivery rate of 35 percent of all babies in the early 1970's had
decreased to 6 percent by the early 1980's. This trend is a direct
result of several studies indicating that babies subject to difficult

forceps delivery may be more prone to birth trauma and asphyxia. Some babies can fit marginally well through the pelvis if assisted with forceps. But rather than subject them to a potentially traumatic vaginal birth, obstetricians are appropriately doing caesarean sections.

Babies born now may actually be bigger than they were in the 1950's and 1960's. In those decades it was common practice to limit maternal weight gain to fifteen pounds. The current recommendation for women of average height and weight is on the order of thirty to thirty-five pounds. While it might seem an easy matter to compare average weights of babies from year to year, it is not as straightforward as it might appear. Nevertheless, it appears that birth weights may have increased over the years. Even an average gain of only a few ounces could have a profound effect on the percentage of babies too large to fit.

CAN I LABOR IF I HAVE HAD A PREVIOUS CAESAREAN DELIVERY?

Repeat caesarean sections are a significant contributor to the rise in caesarean section rates and is the one indication that can be significantly altered. At the turn of the century, when caesarean sections were first done safely, the classical incisions that were common at that time occasionally ruptured with subsequent pregnancies. As a result, obstetricians felt that once the uterus had a through-and-through scar, it was so weakened that subsequent labor was not safe. In the years since, with the widespread preference for the lower cervical transverse incision, the dictum *Once a section, always a section* simply has not been borne out in studies examining the safety of labor following caesarean section.

A uterine rupture consists of a breach in both the uterine wall and the fetal membranes so that the fetus is actually in direct contact with maternal abdominal organs. A uterine dehiscence involves only a defect in the uterus; the amniotic membranes are still intact. This distinction is critical, although in the literature it is sometimes blurred. Early in my training, I noted that women did not seem to have any difficulty laboring after prior caesarean section. I also noticed that a significant number of women undergoing elective repeat caesarean section had defects in the walls of the uterus. It is clear to me now that many women can labor quite normally even with a defect in the uterus provided that the fetal membranes remain intact. This view is well supported by the medical literature.

Labor after prior caesarean section is so safe that medical evidence is not able to demonstrate convincingly that there is any increased risk to the mother or fetus over that of elective repeat caesarean section. Currently, the American College of Obstetrics and Gynecology suggests that a trial of labor may be appropriate in interested women who have had up to two prior caesarean sections. They provide some guidelines that specify that the previous incision had to be the lower cervical transverse type and that repeat caesarean section should be able to be accomplished within thirty minutes, if needed. The College also points out that studies have shown that there is no increased risk for these patients with the use of Pitocin to strengthen contractions or epidural anesthesia for pain relief.

Roughly three out of four women undergoing labor after caesarean section are able to deliver vaginally. These women benefit from less postpartum pain. They go home with their babies significantly sooner, and they are also spared the chance of complications following caesarean birth. Even so, some doctors may hesitate to recommend labor for women with a previous well-documented diagnosis of cephalopelvic disproportion. Although we often encourage labor for this group as well, it seems that these women in particular might have a lower success rate due to the likelihood of a second diagnosis of cephalopelvic disproportion.

WHAT IF MY BABY IS BREECH?

Three to 4 percent of babies at term are in the breech position; that is, they are bottom down. Of this proportion, 60 percent are frank breeches. This means that their legs are sharply flexed at the hips so that their feet are up by their head. Complete breeches are sitting so that their feet are level with their buttocks at the cervix. The third type of breech is a footling breech, with one or both feet leading the way.

Although relatively rare, breech presentation is an important reason for caesarean section. Twenty years ago, roughly 10 percent of breeches underwent operative delivery; the corresponding figure in the mid-1980's is roughly 80 percent to 90 percent. This change in practice has come from numerous studies in the intervening time that seem to show a significantly increased risk for many aspects of labor and delivery in the breech presentation. Unfortunately, studies that lead to statistically valid and meaningful conclusions are extremely difficult to perform on "uncontrolled" human subjects laboring in a wide variety of circumstances. The available data bode poorly, however, for breeches, with mortality rates exceeding head-down babies delivered vaginally by two to five times. What's worse, the incidence of damaged babies delivered as vaginal breeches have been reported to be as high as 16 percent. While this number is high, it probably does not reflect the outcome that can be expected with current obstetric practice. Even so, the consensus is that the breech position is a relatively high-risk presentation.

Much of the difficulty in breech births stems from the fact that the biggest part of the baby, the head, comes last. As a result, the head can get stuck, the umbilical cord is more apt to be compressed, and the spinal column is more likely to be bent dangerously backward. Many obstetricians, myself included, will perform a caesarean section for breech at the mother's request whatever the individual guidelines. This is because when things go wrong during labor with breeches, they often do so suddenly and seriously. An obstetrician is never sure that a breech will deliver without difficulty no matter how big or small the baby is until the baby is in the nursery.

The breech dilemma exemplifies the complexity of the risk-benefit analysis that obstetricians often face. The maternal mortality and complication rate is higher with caesarean section than with vaginal delivery. Yet, for many breech babies, caesarean section is clearly safer. When faced with the choice of increased risk to themselves versus increased risk to the baby, most mothers choose to assume the dangers (albeit relatively small) themselves. This is a striking demonstration of the selflessness that we associate with motherhood.

Is there any subgroup of breech fetuses in which vaginal birth is as safe as caesarean birth? The medical literature suggests that properly screened breech fetuses can deliver with a high degree of safety through the vagina and with greatly reduced pain and complications for the mother. Factors that are often considered in determining whether a vaginal birth is likely to be safe include the type of breech, the estimated fetal weight, the progress in labor, and estimated pelvic size. With careful screening, some breech babies can be delivered safely. In decades past, the great majority of breeches had no problem during vaginal delivery.

WHAT ABOUT FETAL INTOLERANCE TO LABOR?

In about one or two out of a hundred births, the soon-to-be-born infant experiences intolerance to labor requiring prompt intervention. Among mothers with medical problems, this rate may be somewhat higher. Difficulties during labor will result in an inadequate supply of oxygen to a variety of organs including the baby's brain. When your doctor advises you that your fetus is probably not getting enough oxygen to its brain, a caesarean section is the best course of action. It is worth emphasizing that fetal intolerance to labor is uncommon and that emergency caesarean sections are the exception rather than the rule.

WHAT ARE OTHER REASONS FOR CAESAREAN BIRTH?

There are a variety of other reasons to do caesarean sections. One such indication is that of placenta previa, the abnormal implantation of the placenta near the cervix. Another indication for caesarean section is multiple gestation. One to 2 percent of the general population has twins; this number is higher for those on fertility drugs. Twins have a higher incidence of both fetal distress and breech presentations, so they often need to be delivered by caesarean section.

Chapter Ten

CAESAREAN BIRTH

WAS JULIUS CAESAR DELIVERED BY CAESAREAN?

Contrary to popular belief, the caesarean section was not named after Julius Caesar, nor was it the route of his birth. Indeed, the first successful caesarean section on a living woman did not occur until the beginning of the nineteenth century. The name of the operation is thought to come from the Latin verb "to cut," or *caedere*. In Roman times the operation was used to remove a dead baby from a dead mother prior to burial.

This operation had a greater than 50 percent mortality rate until the 1880's, and then it was used only as a last resort to save the mother's life. Improvements in surgical technique, anesthesia, blood banking, and antimicrobial therapy over the past hundred years have reduced the risk so much that caesarean section can now be safely undertaken to benefit the unborn baby.

HOW WILL I BE PREPARED FOR SURGERY?

Preparation for the caesarean section is somewhat different than for a vaginal birth. First, an intravenous line (IV) is inserted into a vein in your arm. Some hospitals have these placed in all laboring patients whether or not a caesarean section is anticipated. You certainly can decline if it is being offered to you routinely, without a specific reason. The IV itself consists of a needle within a hollow plastic tube. The needle is used to guide the hollow tube into the vein and is then removed, leaving the soft, flexible plastic tube in place. This tube is then taped to your skin and connected to a bottle containing sterile water with sugar and salts added in various quantities.

The IV serves several purposes. First, it permits rapid access to your bloodstream for the administration of a wide variety of medications that may be needed in the course of surgery. Second, the IV permits rapid replacement of fluid lost during surgery. Third, in the event that you need a blood transfusion, the IV is already in place. Finally, the IV will provide you with badly needed fluid in the early postoperative period when you may not be able to eat.

In preparation for surgery, a small sample of your blood is matched with blood available in the hospital in case you need a transfusion. A hollow plastic tube called a Foley catheter is then placed through your urethra (urinary hole) into the bladder. This prevents urine from building up in your bladder during the course of surgery and thereby reduces the chance that the bladder will be damaged during the operation.

You are then moved into the operating room, which in most hospitals is contained within the delivery suite. If you are going to receive either an epidural or a spinal anesthetic, it is administered at this time. Your abdomen is thoroughly washed, usually with Betadine, an iodine solution. Your doctor and the assistant then cover you with a series of sterile drapes.

CAN I STAY AWAKE FOR MY BIRTH IF I HAVE A CAESAREAN SECTION?

Yes, under most circumstances. Regional anesthesia, with which you stay awake during surgery, includes two different techniques, the spinal and the epidural. General anesthesia involves putting you to sleep for surgery. The one type of anesthetic that is almost never used anymore for such surgery is the local. A local anesthetic is injected directly into the incision site and provides only limited pain relief. For this reason, regional or general anesthesia are preferred.

A versatile method of delivering anesthesia, the lumbar epidural, can be used with good result to provide anesthesia for caesarean birth, no matter what type of incision your doctor chooses. If the epidural catheter is already in place from labor, you can be redosed with a larger amount of anesthetic, appropriate for surgery. If the tube is not in place, a catheter can be inserted or, more commonly, a single dose of medicine can be injected into the epidural space.

The injection of a narcotic such as morphine into the catheter at the end of surgery is a significant recent development in obstetric anesthesia. A small dose of morphine in the epidural space can provide twelve to sixteen hours of pain relief at the incision. This frees you from the need for pain shots and, since less drug is used, tends to result in fewer side effects, such as nausea and sedation, than the more common injections. Freedom from incision pain with the added feature of being wide-awake are the considerable advantages of this method.

There are some drawbacks to using the epidural for caesarean birth. First, it requires ten to twenty minutes or so to take full effect and, as a result, is unsuitable for an emergency delivery. Second, the pain relief afforded is not total. That is, you can occasionally feel uncomfortable pressure during surgery. If the discomfort becomes too great, the epidural can be supplemented with intravenous narcotics once the baby is born. Also, epidurals are occasionally spotty, that is, they do not provide anesthesia throughout the field of surgery. When this occurs, the condition may be corrected by a change in your position along with a redose of the epidural. In rare instances, a general anesthetic must be given if the epidural proves unsatisfactory. To avoid unanticipated spottiness in pain relief, the region of the abdomen in which the surgery will take place is always carefully tested for sensation by both the anesthesiologist and your obstetrician.

Risks of a lumbar epidural for caesarean section are the same as for labor and have already been discussed (see Chapter Seven). The advantages are the low probability of a spinal headache, your being awake for the birth of your baby, and the opportunity to have anesthetic injected directly into the epidural space. Most hospitals and physicians will encourage the father to be present at the birth when you are awake. This allows him to be an active participant and provide support during delivery.

In the spinal method of administering anesthesia for caesarean section, a needle significantly smaller than the epidural needle is used to puncture the fluid-filled sac containing your spinal nerves. A small amount of anesthetic is injected directly into this sac. While the spinal and epidural each involve injecting anesthetic into the back with a needle, there are significant differences between the two methods.

With the spinal, the onset of pain relief is much faster, generally in three to five minutes rather than the ten to twenty minutes for the epidural. Also, the quality of pain relief tends to be somewhat better than for the epidural, although the latter is adequate in most instances. With spinals, there is much less variation in the quality of numbness throughout the operative field. Finally, significantly less medication is used. This is not an important advantage except for the possibility of an unrecognized wet tap during an epidural. It would be undesirable to inject the larger amount of medication used for an epidural into the place where the spinal anesthetic is injected.

The risks of the spinal mimic those of the epidural. The possibility of low blood pressure, inadequate distribution of numbness, and intravascular injection all exist. The spinal, however, has a slightly higher chance of leaving the patient with a headache. As with the epidural, you are awake for the surgery and the father is often welcome in the operating room.

Back pain following caesarean section is quite common. Patients logically enough link their new back pain with their recent injections. This discomfort is usually the result of lying flat on your back for several hours during the surgery and recovery period. With the numbness from the anesthesia, it is difficult to know what is the most comfortable position during surgery, so the back muscles are often somewhat strained. A heating pad and the passage of time will help this discomfort, which can also occur following general anesthesia.

One final note about spinals and epidurals. Because of a potential drop in blood pressure, the three- to twenty-minute delay required in waiting for them to work, and their less-than-perfect reliability, these methods are not suitable when an emergency caesarean section is needed. Under these circumstances a delay of just a few minutes while waiting for the anesthetic to work may be ill-advised.

It is a memorable experience to perform surgery on a woman who is awake. We talk to you to let you know how things are going. While your husband is asked to sit by your side, more often than not dads stand and peer over the drapes to see better. With the birth of the baby you can hear the first cry, and we usually hold your newborn over the drapes so that you get a quick look also.

WHAT IF I HAVE TO GO TO SLEEP FOR THE DELIVERY?

In current practice, the general anesthetic used for a caesarean section is almost as safe for you and your baby as is the epidural and spinal. The mother-to-be is given thiopental to induce unconsciousness. Within seconds, this drug is followed by a short-acting paralyzing agent injected intravenously. Once paralyzed, you stop breathing on your own, and this function is taken over for you by the anesthesiologist, who holds a mask over your nose and mouth. The air that you breathe through the mask contains oxygen and some anesthetic gas such as Forane to help provide additional pain relief. Within another half-minute, the anesthesiologist inserts a hollow, plastic breathing tube called an endotracheal tube through your mouth into the windpipe. He then inflates a small balloon surrounding the end of the tube within the windpipe to ensure an airtight seal. During general anesthesia, the anesthesiologist monitors you by a continuous cardiogram and by watching your blood pressure, pulse, and the color of skin and nail beds.

While there are a variety of complications from general anesthesia, the one that concerns us is aspiration. This occurs when your stomach contents are inhaled into your airways. A potentially dangerous pneumonia can result. When you are awake, the valve at the top of your windpipe is quite effective in reflexively keeping food out of the windpipe. During the unconsciousness experienced with general anesthesia, your normal reflexes are blocked. This can lead to problems if you regurgitate with a full stomach.

The key to reducing the problems caused by aspiration is to reduce the chances of it occurring rather than try to treat it once it has happened. This can be done in several ways. Reduction of oral intake is the first line of defense. For elective or scheduled surgery, you are asked not to eat or drink anything for eight hours prior to the operation (including liquids such as coffee or water). But there are many caesarean procedures that cannot be scheduled because the need for them becomes clear only after you are well advanced in labor. As soon as your doctor suspects that a caesarean section may be required, he will ask you not to eat or drink anything further during the labor. Usually, this is within a few hours or minutes of the anticipated surgery. This is one of the reasons that many doctors prefer laboring patients to limit their oral intake to clear liquids such as water or jello in the event that they might need surgery and general anesthesia. Aspiration is also a risk during epidural and spinal anesthesia, although a much smaller risk because you are awake.

Reduction of stomach acidity before surgery is another way to reduce the dangers of aspiration. Many anesthesiologists are fond of giving a foul-tasting liquid antacid immediately before surgery. This will reduce the acidity of your stomach contents and may reduce the amount of lung irritation in the event that aspiration occurs. This step is not always practical if you need an emergency caesarean section.

Administration of a paralyzing agent is routine during general anesthesia for caesarean sections. While this sounds dramatic, it has real merit. When you are paralyzed, you cannot contract the abdominal wall muscles and as a result are unable to regurgitate. This also aids the surgeon in relaxing the abdominal walls. The disadvantage is that you cannot breathe on your own. This is not really a disadvantage for the anesthesiologist, since you do not breathe as reliably under general anesthesia anyway and you always need close attention. The anesthesiologist merely takes over your breathing, either manually—by squeezing a bag—or with a respirator.

Finally, insertion of an endotracheal tube is the ultimate defense against aspiration. The tube-balloon combination makes an airtight passageway between the opening of the windpipe and your mouth. That is, the endotracheal tube provides air to the windpipe while the balloon acts to seal off the rest of the passageway. Even if you do regurgitate, the solids or liquids in your mouth are denied access to the windpipe. The endotracheal tube is not removed until you are awake enough to pull it out yourself, thereby assuring that your gag reflex has returned. The endotracheal tube is responsible for the occasional sore throat after surgery. Also, on rare occasions, a tooth may be chipped as the tube is inserted.

General anesthesia can be frightening because, unlike with regional anesthesia, patients are actually unconscious and cannot monitor what is going on around them. Of course, it carries the additional disadvantage of preventing you from enjoying your newborn's first moments of life. However, there are several important advantages of this method. First, the pain relief is immediate and total within sixty seconds of the first injection of drug. Second, the method has virtually 100 percent reliability. It works the first time without the need for a redose or the use of a different method, as may be the case with epidural and spinal anesthetics. Also, it rarely causes a fall in blood pressure, as do the other options.

Some women at time of delivery who have not had an epidural and request pain relief late in labor will be given nitrous oxide, or

laughing gas, by their physician. This gas is not a general anesthetic. Since you do not become unconscious with nitrous oxide,
you are fully able to protect your airway and are therefore not at
increased risk of inhaling solids or liquids into your lungs.

What about my baby? When you receive a general anesthetic
for caesarean delivery, babies born within ten minutes after the
initiation of such anesthesia are rarely sleepy. The average time of
delivery falls well within this time. That is why you are prepped
and draped in advance of the general anesthetic. On those occasions when the baby is somewhat sleepy because he absorbed some
of the drugs given to you, he usually wakes up rather promptly. In
extreme cases, the newborn will need assistance breathing. Since
some neonates require assistance in breathing for other reasons,
the hospital staff is well prepared to provide this service. The
paralytic agent given to you is metabolized rapidly and does not
cross the placenta to the baby in significant amounts.

HOW DOES MY BABY GET DELIVERED?

After the drapes are in position, the various equipment stands are
moved into place and the operating lights are adjusted. You will
often hear a high-pitched sound of the suction equipment used in
the operation. Throughout the course of the surgery, the anesthesiologist sits close to you, checking your blood pressure and other
vital signs every five minutes or so. When your doctor is ready to
proceed, he will gently pinch your skin at the site of the incision to
confirm that the anesthetic is effective. At this point, your partner, if he wishes to, is brought into the operating room and seated
beside you. He is separated from the operating field by a sterile
drape that is maintained above eye level. Many fathers stand and
watch the surgery when they sense that their baby is about to be
born.

There are four basic parts to the operation: making the abdominal incision, making the uterine incisions, delivering the baby,
and closing the wound. Abdominal wall incisions are commonly
vertical or horizontal. The vertical incision is made through the

entire thickness of the abdominal wall. This generally leaves a vertical midline scar between the pubic hairline and the belly button. It takes the shortest time and results in slightly less bleeding than the horizontal incision, or bikini-cut. Also, it can provide better access to the baby for your doctor than the horizontal incision. During emergency surgery when every minute is important, a vertical incision is most commonly made. Occasionally it is done for other reasons, such as the size or position of the baby. Such incisions are often performed for breech babies and anatomical reasons such as fibroids (common outgrowths of muscle on the uterus), low implantation of the placenta, or the presence of large, obstructing veins.

The two types of horizontal incisions, the Pfannenstiel and Mallard, are typically made at the level of your pubic hair line. They are preferable from a cosmetic viewpoint since your scar is obscured by the pubic hairs; few bikinis fail to cover the scar. After the skin and tough underlying tissue, called fascia, are incised, the large muscles of the abdominal wall are encountered. In a Pfannenstiel incision, the muscles are separated vertically in the middle and then retracted. With the Mallard incision, the muscles are actually cut halfway across. Both methods provide adequate room and comparable rates of healing, and the decision as to which one to use is largely the personal preference of the surgeon.

After the muscles have been breached, the abdomen is entered by gently cutting the thin lining of the abdominal cavity known as peritoneum. The type of abdominal wall incision is irrelevant to the next steps. Your doctor reaches in and directly examines the uterus in order to determine better the position and the size of the baby. Your bladder, which covers the lower portion of the uterus, is partially moved away from the uterus wall and retracted out of the way.

There are several types of uterine incisions. The most common one is known as the lower cervical transverse incision and is a horizontal cut in the lower part of the uterus. This technique is thought to leave the strongest scar and is most suitable to withstand labor in subsequent pregnancies. Occasionally a vertical incision has to be made on the uterus because of the baby's position or the woman's anatomy. Your obstetrician will generally prefer to do bikini cuts on the skin and horizontal incisions on the uterus. This combines the best cosmetic result with the most flexibility in terms of labor during subsequent pregnancies.

Once the uterus is open, the baby is ready for delivery. Your obstetrician simply reaches in and guides the head (or buttocks, in the case of a breech) through the incision as his assistant gently presses down on the top of the uterus. The mucus in the baby's mouth and nose are sucked out and the umbilical cord is clamped and cut. If you are awake, you are shown your baby and can touch him with your hand.

Following birth, the placenta is removed and the last step, closing the abdomen, is begun. The uterine incision is generally closed in two separate suture layers. We then commonly sew the thin lining of the abdomen (peritoneum) back together, although not always because this layer heals so quickly even without stitches. The strength of the repair of the next layer, the fascia, determines the strength of the entire wound closure since this is by far the strongest tissue in the abdominal wall. Occasionally sutures are placed in the fatty tissue under the skin. The skin itself is then closed. We use dissolving sutures throughout the procedure. The sutures dissolve slowly as your wound gathers strength. It is thought that this practice results in less internal scar tissue formation.

The least important tissue layer, the skin, attracts the most attention because it is the only part of the wound that you can see. In fact, as long as the underlying abdominal tissues are closed, the skin will invariably heal, regardless of whether it is sutured shut or not. Of course, for aesthetic reasons we always close the skin, as long as there is no serious underlying infection.

There are several ways to accomplish this. The first is to put in several dozen stitches of nonabsorbable suture. These are removed five to six days following surgery. An alternative is to place dissolving sutures immediately under the skin. These sutures cannot be seen and do not need to be removed.

The most commonly used method is to close the skin with steel staples. This has several advantages. Stainless steel generally causes less inflammation when in contact with the skin than the various types of suture materials and, as a result, may leave a smaller scar. This type of closure is significantly faster than suturing. Moreover, it is less uncomfortable to have the staples removed than to have nonabsorbable sutures removed. The staples are generally removed on the third or fourth postoperative day. The procedure is surprisingly fast and causes little discomfort.

After the staples are removed, the doctor will often place strips of a special surgical tape across the incision to help keep the edges together. Neither the staples nor the tape keeps the wound intact. What holds it together are the sutures in the fascia, which are deep within and which are not removed. The special skin tapes can be removed at home seven days after discharge.

The caesarean section itself takes about forty-five minutes. It requires five to ten minutes to make the incision and thirty minutes to repair it. If you have had a previous caesarean section, it will often take somewhat longer. Repeat operations are more difficult due to the buildup of scar tissue.

WHEN CAN I EAT AFTER SURGERY?

Physicians vary somewhat on when they will allow you to eat. Sometimes we start you on clear liquids right away; on occasion we will have you wait several days until you are passing gas from the rectum. In any event, your intestines take a few days to recover their full function, and you may be somewhat prone to nausea during this time. Following the anesthesia for surgery, the intestines' ability to move liquids and solids downstream is diminished. As a result, anything you eat or drink does not move down the gastrointestinal tract properly and instead tends to back up. This may lead to nausea and vomiting in severe cases and is the most important reason why some doctors limit oral intake. Even without any backup problem, you may have nausea. Both the anesthetic and the narcotic pain medications given after surgery can cause an upset stomach.

When the small intestine is in the process of recovering its function, it makes audible gurgling sounds. If these sounds are reasonably normal on the second or third day, most physicians will advance the diet. The large intestine is usually the last part of the bowel to recover full function. This is marked by the passage of rectal gas and can occur as soon as the third day after surgery, though often it takes longer.

As the intestines recover from surgery, you might experience cramps known as gas pain. This discomfort can rival the incision pain. Since the large intestine is the last to work after surgery, the cramps come from the small intestine trying to push material downstream into the unyielding large bowel. No medicine or activity will do much to hasten recovery of your bowel. Generally your gas pain and some distention of the abdomen is worst from post-op day two to day four. Once you pass gas out of the rectum, the pain usually resolves in twenty-four hours. Pain medicine may relieve some of your discomfort.

Passing gas is, of course, a good omen for your first bowel movement after surgery, which is often small and loose. Full return of bowel function varies greatly from patient to patient. Occasionally a week goes by before you have your first bowel movement, although gas is usually passed before this point. Once in a while, we will send you home before your first bowel movement, but usually not before you pass gas.

WHEN CAN MY IV AND FOLEY CATHETER COME OUT?

Intravenous fluids speed your recovery by assuring proper fluid intake while you are unable to drink. You may find it trying despite its benefits. While it is not uncomfortable, it is an inconvenience to be physically connected to plastic tubing, a bottle, and a steel pole. As long as you are not nauseated and can keep down liquids, the IV is usually removed following the first day or so. This procedure takes a few seconds and does not hurt.

If you require antibiotics for a postoperative infection, the IV will remain in place for several days longer than ordinary. Also, the IV will be reinserted in a different location every two or three days to avoid an inflammation that could temporarily close off the vein.

Following surgery, the Foley catheter is often allowed to stay in place for twenty-four hours. You can usually tolerate this bladder tube quite well. On the plus side, you do not have to get out of bed to urinate every few hours on the first day after surgery. However, the longer the catheter remains in, the greater the chance of bladder infection, although after only twenty-four hours this is not a major concern. Removing the Foley takes a moment and is not uncomfortable. You may have some difficulty urinating at first, and the Foley might have to be replaced for a day or two. Due to a buildup of fluid during pregnancy, you might find that you are urinating much more than usual during the week after the birth of your baby.

HOW MUCH PAIN WILL I HAVE?

The pain of the incision is significant for the first several days but decreases with each passing day. During this period, when you are not taking medicine by mouth, narcotic injections are given every three or four hours, at your request. Commonly used drugs are Demerol, Dilaudid, or morphine; all are narcotics and are interchangeable. If one drug does not agree with you, an alternative can be tried. When you are taking food by mouth, pain pills are provided. Unfortunately all narcotic pain medication tends to promote constipation.

A new technique of narcotic administration that allows patients to administer their own pain relief is becoming widely available and will help make the postoperative period more comfortable. These special narcotic infusion pumps allow patients to control the infusion of pain medication through their intravenous lines. Studies have shown that when patients are given the opportunity to regulate their own infusion, they achieve better pain relief and actually use less drug in comparison with the injection given by the nurse every few hours. You will probably be less sedated with this method and make a speedier recovery. It also spares you the need for unpleasant injections of narcotics. The machines have special lock buttons that allow your doctor to set a maximum amount of drug to be given in any period of time.

Another technique of postoperative pain relief that has been recently developed is that of epidural analgesia. This involves infusing narcotics through the epidural catheter. The advantage is that high concentrations of drugs are delivered close to the pain-sensing nerves while the total dose of drug is quite small. Epidural analgesia provides incomparable pain relief with little or none of the nausea and sedation associated with narcotics. Of course, this method is available only to those with an epidural catheter in place.

WHEN CAN I GET UP? WHEN CAN I SEE MY BABY?

You will be encouraged to sit up in bed and walk as soon as possible, since this hastens all aspects of recovery. Your doctor and nurses know that movement during the first few days is rather uncomfortable. Yet not only is movement encouraged, so is deep breathing and coughing. While you might fear that hard coughing may cause some injury, this is not the case. The more active you are, the faster you will leave the hospital.

You will be quite uncomfortable on the delivery day and may have less energy to be with your baby. However, rooming in is still possible and so is nursing. If you want to, you will be encouraged to nurse immediately following surgery. None of the drugs commonly given during or after the surgery will interfere with breast-feeding.

WHAT ARE THE DANGERS OF A CAESAREAN SECTION?

Although often done to minimize risk for the baby, caesarean section poses significant risks to your health. The risk of maternal death due to caesarean birth from nonanesthetic-related causes generally ranges from roughly 1 per 2,000 operations undertaken during labor to 1 in 5,000 operations undertaken before the onset of labor. The generally accepted maternal mortality rate of vaginal births is 1 per 10,000. The statistics may be misleading, since many of the mothers who die belong to a small fraction of the population who are severely ill at the time of the operation. Indeed, the illness that placed the women at increased surgical risk is often the same condition that required the operation in the first place. In one study reported in the medical literature, more than ten thousand caesarean births were performed without a single maternal death. Most authorities agree, however, that the maternal risk of death from caesarean birth is two to five times greater than it is from vaginal delivery.

A bigger problem than the risk of maternal death is the higher rate of complications following caesarean section compared to the rate associated with vaginal birth. The more common problems are reviewed below. These include infection, damage to adjacent organs, blood clots, and blood loss. Even without any complications, it takes significantly longer to recover from a caesarean section than from a vaginal delivery.

Factors that predispose a patient to postpartum endometritis, or infection of the uterine lining, include prolonged rupture of membranes (anything over three hours, in some studies), long labor, operating time of more than one hour, and low socioeconomic class of the patient. In some studies, womb infections have resulted in 40 percent of all women undergoing caesarean birth. This complication is not as bad as it sounds, since the vast majority of these infections respond readily to antibiotics.

Caesarean section predisposes a woman to infection of the uterus because contact is inevitably made with the cervix and upper vagina, portions of the body that cannot be meaningfully cleansed prior to surgery. This tends to increase the number of bacteria present within the womb following either rupture of membranes or labor. Though the body can ably fight off a few bacteria, the probability of infection rises with the number of bacteria present. Also, the tissue damage inherent in surgery provides ideal conditions for bacterial growth.

The most common symptom of postpartum endometritis is a fever that persists to the third or fourth day after surgery. Other symptoms include an unusually tender uterus or a malodorous vaginal discharge, although this latter condition is rare. If your obstetrician suspects that you have an infection, he will usually prescribe intravenous antibiotics for several days until the fever drops. While a womb infection is a relatively common complication of caesarean birth, it is usually not difficult to treat.

Before leaving the subject of infections, a word about fevers is in order. In general, any temperature over 99.4 degrees is considered abnormal, although many medical organizations do not regard temperatures under 100.4 as noteworthy. With any type of infection, including postpartum endometritis, it is common for your temperature to vary greatly. At some points during the day it may even be normal. To evaluate the antibiotic treatment, your doctor will look for the highest temperature in a twenty-four-hour period and compare it to that of the previous day. As long as the maximum temperature drops from one day to the next, we believe that the treatment is working. Once the temperature has been continuously normal for one to two days, you may be switched to oral antibiotics and discharged from the hospital. After you go home, your obstetrician may have you check your temperature periodically for a few days to be sure that the fever does not return with the modification in therapy.

Steps can be readily taken to reduce the likelihood of endometritis following caesarean section. One or more doses of antibiotics, for example, can be given to you at the time of surgery and immediately thereafter. This practice has been shown to reduce significantly the incidence of postoperative fever attributable to endometritis. A common practice is for the antibiotics to be given immediately following delivery of the baby. This enables the pediatrician to obtain bacterial cultures on the newborn if he suspects infection, without concern that the antibiotics given you will interfere with the tests for infection on your infant.

The wound itself can get infected, although this is much less common than endometritis. Fever, a significant increase in redness and pain around the incision, and the formation of pus all suggest that a wound infection may be developing. You will be treated with antibiotics as described above. In addition, the skin edges might have to be separated to allow the underlying pus to drain. This sounds much worse that it is because the wound will heal just as well after the temporary delay of waiting for the infection to be treated.

As with any surgery, adjacent organs can occasionally be damaged in the course of an operation. This risk tends to increase with the presence of prior abdominal surgery or the delivery of a baby far down in the birth canal. The structure most commonly injured during surgery is the bladder, as it lies immediately in front of the uterus. Other structures at risk include the intestines, the urine tubes leading to the bladder, and large blood vessels. Most damage is mild in nature and is easily repaired at the time of surgery without significant additional hardship for you. Occasionally the damage can be more severe, necessitating subsequent operations to repair. Fortunately, such complications are infrequent.

Potentially serious blood clots can occur in the deep leg veins (not the superficial varicose veins). These clots can grow and then break off, posing a threat of severe damage to the lungs. Significant blood clots in the legs are also uncommon and respond well to intravenous blood thinner (heparin). Early walking following surgery tends to help keep the blood in the veins circulating and reduces the chance of blood clots forming.

While the average vaginal birth involves the loss of one pint of blood, twice this amount is lost during the average caesarean birth. You normally add at least a unit of blood to your body over the course of pregnancy. This allows you to tolerate blood loss better than nonpregnant people. Furthermore, as new mothers are mostly young and healthy, blood transfusions are generally not considered until you have lost half of the blood in your body. Even with caesarean birth, this is a relatively unusual problem, although by no means rare. Obstetricians try not to transfuse you unless it is absolutely necessary to preserve your health. Your doctor would rather have you take iron tablets for three months after the delivery than transfuse. To help minimize your need for transfusion, your blood count is checked in the prenatal period so that you can be prescribed the appropriate amount of iron in preparation for birth.

What are the risks of a blood transfusion? The most basic problems are allergic reactions and the spread of infectious diseases. Immediate reactions to blood products generally occur in 5 percent of the population and range from itching, rashes, and fever to more severe allergic symptoms. Blood incompatibility resulting in a severe allergic reaction is rare with current blood-banking techniques. Longer-term allergic reactions can occur when you receive several blood transfusions at different points in your life. The foreign proteins on the blood cells in the first transfusion can prime your immune system to respond if you are exposed to those proteins again in another blood transfusion. The nature of these delayed allergic reactions is highly variable and is only a consideration for those who have received blood in the past.

A common concern of patients who receive blood transfusions is the risk of acquiring an infectious disease, particularly AIDS. The risk is related to blood-banking procedures. Blood can be obtained from either volunteer donors or from those who are paid to donate. In general, paid donors tend to be people who need money rather badly. As a result, a disproportionate number of substance abusers contribute blood to these blood collection agencies, in comparison to people who donate blood. Paid-donor blood is well known to have a higher incidence of infectious-disease agents than volunteer-donor blood. Also, the incidence of disease in volunteer blood varies substantially with the background of the volunteers. As a result, the probability of acquiring an infectious disease can vary considerably among various communities, depending on the underlying prevalence of a particular disease.

An additional consideration is the availability of a screening test for the infectious agent. For instance, all blood banks screen every unit of blood for the virus that causes hepatitis B, a potentially fatal illness. While 1 percent of the population carries this virus and is potentially infectious, the risk to blood recipients is much lower because of the screening test. One suburban blood-bank director advised me that out of 90,000 transfused units in one year in his system, two people acquired hepatitis B. Blood is also routinely screened for syphilis and AIDS. A new test for hepatitis C is now being widely used, which makes the blood supply safer than ever before.

One issue that is frequently raised by patients is their desire to designate specific donors for their transfusions. Unfortunately, under pressure, relatives might donate blood without confessing that they have had a socially embarrassing disease such as syphilis or AIDS. In fact, some studies have demonstrated that blood from designated donors is somewhat more likely to carry disease than blood from anonymous donors.

Another issue that occasionally arises is the possibility of auto-donation. For some elective surgeries you can donate a unit of blood two weeks in advance of surgery. The blood can be stored while your body replenishes its supply. Unfortunately, this is not applicable to most caesarean sections. The majority of caesarean sections are not scheduled, and no one can predict precisely when you will go into labor. If you begin labor too soon after you give blood, you will be relatively short of blood and increase your odds of needing a transfusion. Also, obstetricians rarely transfuse patients unless absolutely necessary and, when they do, they usually administer multiple units—much more than could be safely donated by one person. Finally, many pregnant patients are somewhat anemic in the first place and need all the blood they have. With these limitations in mind, obstetricians will often suggest autodonation for women undergoing scheduled, repeat caesarean sections.

The risks of not receiving a recommended blood transfusion are both complex and serious. First, it is difficult for your doctor to know exactly how much blood you have left after you have hemorrhaged. Second, no one can easily predict how much additional bleeding will occur following birth. Finally, it is difficult to accurately predict at what level of anemia you will suffer heart attacks, brain damage, or kidney death. While obstetricians are reluctant to transfuse, these complications are severe indeed. Again, your doctor will recommend a blood transfusion only when he or she feels the risk of proceeding is less than the risk of withholding the blood.

CAN A CAESAREAN SECTION HARM MY BABY?

In decades past, some elective caesarean sections were performed too early and could well have resulted in the delivery of a premature baby. The most prominent problem among these premature babies is trouble breathing outside the womb, occasionally necessitating a respirator. With the wide availability of ultrasound to assist with gestational age assessment and more careful attention to scheduling repeat caesarean sections closer to the due date, premature delivery is no longer a significant problem.

Another potential adverse effect is known as transient tachypnea of the newborn. While this condition is usually mild and temporary, it can cause the term infant to have some difficulty breathing, manifested by a fast respiratory rate and chest retraction and grunting. This typically clears up without much intervention and with no adverse consequences. Although this can occur following vaginal birth, some physicians think that it is more common following caesarean birth.

Rarely, the fetus will be scratched during the incision into the uterus. In most cases, the wound is slight and heals without medical treatment.

Chapter Eleven

THE NEWBORN

When your baby's head emerges from your body, he may blink and open his eyes. Often, even before the shoulders emerge, the neonate will gasp his first breath or cry. Some babies may not cry for several minutes after birth. I have yet to predict or understand which ones cry and which ones sleep.

In the first few minutes after birth, the umbilical cord will be clamped and cut, and your baby will be dried off and bathed. Most hospitals go to great effort to avoid separating newborns from their parents, particularly in the first few hours of life. When not in your arms, your baby will be wrapped in a blanket and kept in an incubator. Modern incubators use radiant heat so that the baby does not need to be encased in glass. Since newborns lose heat quickly because of a large area of skin relative to their small bodies, hats are often put on them to help keep them warm.

THE FIRST TEST

In our competitive society, where most things seem to be measured and large numbers are usually better than small ones, it should be no surprise that the baby is given a test in the first minute of life. In 1953, a pediatrician, Dr. Virginia Apgar, developed a brief quantifiable physical exam for babies that could be used to guide physicians and nurses in their care of the neonate in his first few minutes of life. It is called an Apgar score, and it is not really a test, but parents often are preoccupied with the numbers it assigns to their baby.

Dr. Apgar designed her exam with very narrow goals in mind. Unfortunately, many people both in and out of the medical profession have misconstrued her intent. They erroneously use the Apgar score as a type of IQ test, or to predict brain damage due to birth trauma. The Apgar score has nothing to do with brain damage, mental retardation, or birth defects. It is meant only to guide medical personnel in intervening on the baby's behalf in the first few minutes of life.

The baby is studied briefly twice, first one minute after birth and then five minutes after birth; a score from zero to ten is given both times. The scoring system consists of five easily observed features of the baby. Each category is assigned a zero, one, or two. The higher the score, the more vigorous the infant. In terms of assessing the overall health of the baby, the five-minute Apgar score is much more important than the one-minute score. Sometimes babies seem to be surprised by their new environment and need a few minutes to perk up.

THE APGAR SCORING SYSTEM

Category	Zero	One	Two
Heart rate	Absent	Below 100	Above 100
Respiration	Absent	Weak	Good, crying
Muscle tone	Limp	Some	Active
Responsiveness	Absent	Some	Active
Color	Blue	Blue in hands, feet only	Pink

A score of seven or above indicates that the infant needs little assistance in adjusting to life outside of the mother. A score of four to six often indicates that the baby may need assistance breathing, if only for a short time. A score of zero to three indicates that the baby is having significant difficulty adjusting to his new environment. Low-scoring babies are often quite ill and may need considerable medical assistance, including a ventilator and medicines administered through IV lines.

Few infants achieve a perfect score at either one or five minutes. Their arms beyond the elbows and their legs beyond their knees are almost always at least somewhat blue, even at five minutes. Also, not all infants cry loudly at birth. Some are content to rest quietly in their swaddling. Regrettably, many new parents are convinced that their baby is not alive until they hear that first cry, no matter what reassurance is provided. For this reason, I find it helpful to hand the baby directly to the parents immediately after birth for at least a brief time so that they can see their new child for themselves. The nurse then "borrows" the baby for a few minutes to dry it off. Very shortly after birth, the nurse will obtain a footprint of the baby and apply identification bracelets. Usually these are plastic bands that attach to an arm and a leg. The footprint is actually an anachronism, since very few babies could be positively identified on the basis of the print alone.

Recently a fellow pediatrician and I were talking about Apgar scoring as we were waiting for a delivery. We both felt oppressed by parents' anxieties over this score. Parents should really ask, "Is my baby healthy, or does he need assistance?" However, they usually ask, "What is his Apgar score?" Some parents want to know why their child does not have a perfect score, even though we rarely give such a score since most babies are a little blue at first. (The British system goes up to eight and does not evaluate color at all.) My colleague told me that for those who ask, he explains that Apgar scores are like bowling or golf. You can bowl a 270 or shoot one over par for the course—wonderful scores but not perfect. In writing about this subject, I realize now that I do not even know the Apgar scores for any of my own children. It never occurred to me to ask. I thought that if they were crying and wiggling within the first five minutes of life, they must be fine.

WHAT IF MY BABY HAS PROBLEMS?

Most babies are healthy at birth and do not require any medical assistance, but sometimes they require some help.

Narcotics given to you, whether given alone or with a general anesthetic, do reach the baby. Generally the doses of narcotics given during labor wear off entirely by the time of birth and are not likely to effect the baby. Occasionally a mother will be given narcotics just before birth and the baby may be sedated. A sedated baby typically has decreased respiratory functions and does not move as much as he might otherwise. First the baby will be given a small shot in the thigh of the drug known as Narcan. This drug reverses the sedative effects of narcotics within seconds. Also, the baby's breathing will be assisted by an oxygen mask that is held over his mouth and nose. This mask has a small bag that the nurse will squeeze to blow air into the baby's lungs until he wakes up. Generally this is necessary for only a few minutes.

When meconium is present at birth, the nurse or physician will quickly examine the infant's windpipe in an effort to determine if meconium is present below the vocal cords. To do this, an endotracheal, or breathing, tube is inserted through the infant's mouth to allow the doctor to see the upper portion of the windpipe. If meconium is present below the vocal cords, a narrow plastic suction tube will be inserted in an effort to remove the material before it moves into the baby's lungs.

There are several facts to keep in mind. First, meconium rarely causes significant difficulty for the infant. In most cases, the amount of meconium taken into the airways is minimal. Second, the medical staff will try to suction the baby's windpipe before the infant has an opportunity to cry vigorously. As a result, the baby will be whisked away from the parents to the corner of the room with the incubator. Usually everything is finished within five minutes so that the parents may then hold the baby. Third, since the baby is unable to make noises with the breathing tube inserted into the windpipe, the parents will not be able to hear him cry. This does not signify a jeopardized baby and is almost always a brief procedure.

WILL MY BABY NEED ANY BLOOD TESTS?

Most states mandate a variety of blood tests for the baby within the first few days of life. Two of the most common tests are chemical screening procedures for phenylketonuria (PKU) and hypothyroidism. Both of these relatively uncommon problems are preventable causes of mental retardation. Many states also mandate an injection of vitamin K within the first day of life. Vitamin K is necessary to help the liver produce clotting proteins; without it, babies tend to bleed. Babies are often low on this vitamin, and there is little harm in injecting a supplementary dose.

A somewhat controversial requirement for hospital births is that babies receive eye drops to prevent gonorrhea. At the turn of the century, gonorrhea eye infections were one of the leading causes of blindness in this country. Since this is such a disaster for an individual, all babies are treated whether or not there is any history or suspicion of maternal gonorrhea. The most commonly used drugs are silver nitrate drops and one of a variety of antibiotics. All of the medications used to prevent gonorrhea of the eyes irritate them for one or two days. As a result, babies occasionally have red eyes associated with a discharge for a few days following birth. Although parents occasionally wish to have the eye drops postponed, the medication needs to be given soon after birth if it is to be effective. The antibiotics most commonly used will also kill chlamydia bacteria that can infect the newborn's eyes.

WHAT ELSE SHOULD I KNOW ABOUT
MY NEW BABY?

The average weight of a newborn infant is seven pounds four ounces. Its average length is twenty inches. Boys tend to weigh somewhat more than girls and tend to be somewhat longer. During the first few days of life, babies lose up to 10 percent of their weight (averaging nine ounces) as they become oriented and learn how to feed. Infants do not know how to suckle efficiently for several days. In the first half day of life, they will be offered water if you are not inclined to breast-feed. During the first two or three days of life, the baby's stools, simply the intestinal secretions that have accumulated over the nine months of the pregnancy, are greenish-black. Gradually, the stools become yellow. During the first thirty days, babies move their bowels one to four times per day, although diarrhea is not uncommon.

Babies are not miniature adults. In particular, their heads are relatively large in proportion to their bodies. Also, the skull bones have not fused and will not close until their first birthday. This feature allows the baby's head to be squeezed into a more suitable shape for passing through the birth canal. Depending on the size of the baby and the passageway, some heads will be more elongated than others. This is known as molding. The head will gradually return to the anticipated spherical shape over a period of days. There may also be some swelling in the baby's scalp as a result of hours of pressure during labor. This, too, will disappear in a day or so and does not represent any damage to the baby.

Occasionally, on the second or third day of life, the baby's skin will assume a yellowish tinge. This mild jaundice is a normal occurrence in the first week and represents an increase in the levels of a substance called bilirubin, one of the breakdown products of red blood cells. Bilirubin in excessive quantities can be toxic to the newborn. If the blood bilirubin becomes too high, the pediatrician will want to keep the baby in the hospital a few extra days for phototherapy treatment. The staff shines an ultraviolet light on the baby to help him eliminate the excess bilirubin. Although parents are often discouraged because they cannot take the baby home when they expected, the jaundice is usually a minor, temporary problem. Also, new techniques are becoming available to allow newborns to be treated at home.

Babies are all born with blue eyes. In those destined to have brown eyes, the color will turn at several months of age. The baby's fine scalp hair will begin to fall out in the second week, to be replaced gradually by coarser, firmer hairs.

Many hospitals will have the nurses paint the inch-long umbilical cord stump with a purple dye to reduce the chance of infection. The clamp left on the cord can be removed after a few days. By the end of the first week the stump is shriveled, often little more than dry black string. The remainder of the stump falls off between seven and eighteen days later.

SHOULD MY BOY GET CIRCUMCISED?

A circumcision is a minor surgical procedure that removes the foreskin covering the penis. Approximately 80 percent of male infants born in this country are circumcised, although this percentage may be dropping. The health benefits of this operation remain open to discussion. The old arguments of improved personal hygiene and reduced chance of penile cancer do not hold up under scientific scrutiny, although there is some suggestion that urinary-tract infection rates may be lower. Many people want their baby to be circumcised for religious or social reasons. For instance, if the father is circumcised, parents will often want the infant circumcised. This is purely a personal decision.

The circumcision itself can be done after twenty-four hours of life, usually before discharge from the hospital. Jaundice and certain anatomical variations in the penis itself will generally cause a postponement in the procedure. The surgery takes three to five minutes and carries unusually low risk. However, as with any surgery, there is always the possibility that the baby may lose enough blood to require a transfusion. Rarely, the circumcision does not achieve the desired results and plastic surgery is subsequently needed if too much skin is removed. Of course, this possibility is a major consideration in the mind of the obstetrician who performs the procedure, so it is a rare problem indeed.

Many doctors are now giving injections of local anesthetic at the base of the penis to ease the discomfort of the procedure.

While not an entirely new idea, this practice has only recently been gaining acceptance. It is both safe and effective.

WHO SHOULD BREAST-FEED?

Breast-feeding has been the subject of intense controversy for many years. Those for and against this practice have been outspoken on the issue. Breast-feeding is probably somewhat healthier for the baby than bottle-feeding, although infants thrive perfectly well on formula. Whether to breast-feed and when to stop are often vexing questions for mothers and are frequently associated with inappropriate feelings of guilt. As with the issues surrounding pain relief during labor, breast-feeding is a highly personal issue.

Working mothers, mothers with twins or other small infants, and mothers with medical problems are often too busy or worn out to devote the extra time and energy required to breast-feed. Some mothers simply do not feel comfortable with breast-feeding. They worry that the baby may be getting too much or too little. In any case, the most important consideration in whether to breast-feed or bottle-feed is your desires. No one benefits if you are pressed into breast-feeding by family members or outsiders. You take the course of action that makes you most comfortable.

IS BREAST-FEEDING BETTER FOR MY BABY THAN BOTTLE-FEEDING?

Each method has its proponents. Breast milk is ideally suited to the neonate's nutritional requirements; presumably time and evolution have resulted in countless modifications in the natural formula. Since human milk contains more calories to the ounce than formula substitutes, breast-fed babies tend to gain weight more rapidly. Furthermore, the nutrients in breast milk tend to be easier to digest than those in formula milk, and therefore stomach and intestinal disturbances tend to be less common in nursed babies. Breast milk does contain maternal antibodies—proteins that might help the baby fend off infection—though this benefit is mainly theoretical and may not make much difference in practice. Finally, breast-feeding is more economical and there is no possibility of improperly prepared or stored food for the baby.

Some studies demonstrate objective improvements in mother-baby interactions when babies are breast-fed. However, it cannot be overemphasized that the mother-infant bond will be strongest if the mother is comfortable with the method that she has chosen for feeding her baby.

Artificial feeding also has its advantages. It may be easier for you to control your weight and body fat merely by regulating the caloric intake if you are not breast-feeding. There is always a ready supply of formula, whereas the quantity of breast milk produced in any given day can vary considerably. Your husband, or anyone else, can just as readily feed the baby, giving you a chance to rest. Finally, working mothers may find breast-feeding to be prohibitively cumbersome and tiring.

HOW DO I NURSE?

As a general rule, breast-feeding is sufficient to provide all of the infant's nutritional needs during the first six months of life. Babies who are put to the breast within the first hour of life seem to have better subsequent success nursing than those infants for whom initial nursing is delayed for several hours. On the first day, the newborn should be allowed to suckle at each breast for five minutes per feeding with the amount of time spent gradually increasing. A demand feeding schedule is the best way to assure both an adequate milk supply and a satisfied, well-nourished infant. This usually leads to more frequent nursing with the best flow of milk.

The amount of breast milk secreted per day varies greatly from woman to woman but averages one-half pint at first. This increases to a pint by the seventh day of breast-feeding and to two pints by two weeks. Immediately after birth, a light yellow watery liquid, called colostrum, is secreted from the nipples. Usually by the third day postpartum colostrum is replaced by milk. As the milk comes in, the breasts become engorged. Although this can be uncomfortable at times, it is short-lived and can be relieved by ice packs and successful nursing. The swelling comes from congestion in the blood vessels of the breast rather than from the milk glands themselves.

Nursing women have clearly increased nutritional requirements. The increased need for food is thought to range from 500 to 1,000 calories per day. Some physicians recommend increased intake of fluids as well, particularly milk and water, although this is not directly related to increased milk production. While it has not been proved, many mothers are convinced that when they eat some foods such as tomatoes and pickles they can make the baby colicky. Generally, milk production will be affected only by extremes in diet (i.e., fewer calories or less fluid).

While nursing, it is helpful to hold the baby in a semi-reclining position, since the baby is less likely to swallow air. The infant should be held so that he has easy access to the nipple without stretching. Also, since the baby knows how to breathe only through the nose immediately after birth, the nursing mother should be sure that the infant has a clear nasal passageway. Since a baby inevitably takes in some air during feeding, he can be made more comfortable after he has had his fill by being placed over your shoulder and by having his back gently tapped. This "burping" of the baby helps him to release air accumulated in the stomach.

WHAT IF I DO NOT WANT TO NURSE?

If you do not want to breast-feed, simply avoid nipple stimulation and wear a tight bra. Significant breast engorgement will typically occur on postpartum days three and four. It can be treated with mild pain relievers and ice packs; it generally goes away within a few days. Many mothers, of course, would like to avoid this uncomfortable period. In the past, estrogen shots were available to suppress lactation and there was an alternative oral medication called Parlodel, but questions have arisen about the safety and effectiveness of both medications. As a result, most doctors no longer prescribe medication to women who choose not to nurse.

A FINAL WORD

As a doctor who deals every day with pregnant and laboring patients, I believe that the medical profession can provide three benefits. Most important, we can give much needed reassurance and emotional support. Relieving the pain of labor is another important service we can provide. Finally, we can intervene on rare occasions where the health of the mother or baby is threatened.

When you enter the hospital, you give up some of your autonomy. This lack of control serves only to increase the anxiety of many mothers entering labor and is precisely the opposite of what we hope to achieve. By providing you with more knowledge about what will be done for you and to you in labor and delivery, I have tried to impart to you a feeling of control. Also, many mothers are too stressed or intimidated to ask questions about what is going on during labor and delivery. I hope this book has answered many of your questions and will encourage you to ask whatever you would like to know during this most exciting and momentous time of your life.

INDEX TO BIRTH DAY!

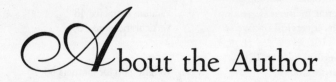bout the Author

Michael D. Benson is an attending obstetrician at Highland Park Hospital, Highland Park, Illinois. He is in practice with two other obstetricians, Dr. Ruth Guth and Dr. Cheryl Perlis. Board certified in Obstetrics and Gynecology, he is a member of Alpha Omega Alpha, a medical honor society and is a lecturer at Northwestern University Medical School.

Dr. Benson has written over 20 medical publications, including five books. Two of these books are for the general population, *Birth Day! The Last 24 Hours of Pregnancy,* and *Coping With Birth Control.* His obstetrical text, *Obstetrical Pearls: A Guide for the Efficient Resident* is in its second edition and has been widely read. It has been translated into Japanese, Indonesian, Spanish, and Portuguese and has also been published in India. His gynecology text, *Gynecologic Pearls: A Guide for the Efficient Resident* has just been published. His current research interest includes adolescent behavior and amniotic fluid embolism, a rare malady of pregnant women.

Dr. Benson lives in Deerfield, Illinois, with his wife Bonnie and three young children.